Helping Your Child Recover
from Sexual Abuse

Helping Your Child Recover
from Sexual Abuse

Caren Adams, M.A.

and

Jennifer Fay, M.A.

Illustrations by A.G. Fawkes

University of Washington Press

Seattle and London

This book was originally published under the title *Never Again: A Parent's Guide to Child Sexual Abuse Recovery* as a project of the Children's Home Society of Washington, Vancouver Branch, Vancouver, Washington. Original publication was funded in part by United Way of the Columbia-Willamette, the Stuart Foundations, Boise Cascade, and private contributors.

Third printing, with updated resource list, 1998
Printed in the United States of America

17   11

University of Washington Press
www.washington.edu/uwpress

Library of Congress Cataloging-in-Publication Data
Adams, Caren, 1946–
    Helping your Child Recover from Sexual Abuse.
    Bibliography: p.
    1. Child molesting—United States. 2. Sexually abused children—Rehabilitation—United States. 3. Sexually abused children—Psychology. I. Fay, Jennifer, 1946–   II. Title.
HQ72.U53A47   1992   362.7'044   88-37877
ISBN-13: 978-0-295-96806-3
ISBN-10: 0-295-96806-0

The paper used in this publication is acid-free and recycled from 10 percent post-consumer and at least 50 percent pre-consumer waste. It meets the minimum requirements of American National Standard for Information Sciences—Permanence of Paper for Printed Library Materials, ANSI Z39.48-1984. ⊗

NEVER AGAIN

> I swore it would never happen
>> to them.
> I was going to make their world safe
> Protect them from the danger I knew.

Never again
> should children be forced to think
> to be equal to those who stand
>> three feet over them
> speak their minds and make them
>> listen.
> Can't they just be children.

Never again
> take for granted
>> a summer's day softness
>> or a neighbor's good will.

Never again
> believe I can keep
> it from happening
> Never again.

—Caren Adams

This book is dedicated to all those parents who are courageously facing this problem.

C.A., Renton, Washington
J.F., Portland, Oregon

Contents

Introduction   xi

Notes on Using this Book   xiii

Acknowledgments   xiv

1. Right Away... "I believe you."   1

The struggle with your own disbelief and the immediate
decisions. How to go back and change immediate responses
you are not happy with. How to act with your child; what to
say. Finding help.

2. The Legal System... "They'll be asking a lot of questions."   19

The range of experiences. Benefits to the child. What makes
the process hard. Helping your child through the interviews
and court. Presenting the outcome to your child.

3. Family and Friends' Responses... "She cares, she just
doesn't understand."   37

The responses of loved ones to the abuse are very important
to your child's well-being. Who to tell, common reactions of
friends and relatives, strategies for responding and helping
the child to understand.

4. Children's Reactions and Everyday Life... "It's okay to be
angry."   49

The difficulties of living with a child on the roller coaster of
recovery. Don't throw out all you know about raising
children. Treat your child as normally as you can. Common
behavior changes and how to respond to them. How to
know that your child is getting better.

5. Grieving. . . **"I'm crying, but I can still take care of you."**   63

In the stress following disclosure of sexual abuse, parents
need to begin to grieve their losses, and help the child to do
that, too. How to find ways to grieve that won't add to your
child's burden. Remembering your own abuse as a child;
taking care of yourself.

6. Rebuilding Self-Esteem. . . **"It wasn't your fault."**   79

Children who have been sexually abused may not feel as
good about themselves as other children. Why children
blame themselves for what happened. How to help your
child regain confidence. The different needs of boys and girls.
Examples of affirmations.

7. Sexuality. . . **"You are still lovable."**   93

Does child sexual abuse affect adult sexuality? Helping your
child to unlearn what the sexual abuse taught. How to deal
with your child's confusions about his or her body.

8. Self-Protection. . . **"Never Again."**   107

Part of recovering from sexual abuse is feeling safe and
feeling in control, and being able to recognize and avoid poor
treatment at the hands of others. How to trust again,
establish privacy and boundaries, and better understand
manipulation. How to teach your child to recognize
behaviors that signal potential sexual abuse. Encouraging
telling.

9. As Children Grow. . . **"We'll need to talk again."**   127

How the meaning of the sexual abuse experience changes as
children grow and mature. Differences for boys and girls.
Typical problems that surface at different ages.

10. Moving on. . . **"It's better now."**   **141**

    Forgiving yourself. How this society lets children down.
    Taking action in the struggle to reduce child abuse. Finding a
    new balance between naive and cynical. Trusting a sunny
    day again. Celebrating with your child.

Selected Resources   **151**

What Is Sexual Abuse?   **155**

Offender Information: "How could he?"   **157**

"One day, when I was cooking spaghetti sauce, my three-year-old daughter matter-of-factly announced that the man next door had given her a cookie and then asked her to pull her pants down. I couldn't believe it. I asked her if she meant Mr. Pomeroy, who has been our neighbor for years. She said yes, and went on to tell me about other 'games' Mr. Pomeroy plays. I didn't want to believe what I was hearing. I felt as though this might be something she imagined, or heard from the other kids or the TV, but, slowly, I began to realize it just might be happening."

"When my son came home from visiting his dad's he was a different five year old. He was withdrawn, he had nightmares and he wet the bed. When the masturbation all the time started, and he was so aggressive that his day care worker told me he couldn't return unless I got him help, I knew I had to do something. After many months seeing a therapist, my son told about sexual abuse by his dad."

"I got this call from my daughter's school. I've never been so shocked. Apparently they had a presentation on personal safety and my daughter told her sixth grade teacher that someone had been 'touching' her. My first reaction was that she just wanted some attention from her teacher—that it couldn't possibly be true."

INTRODUCTION

One day your child says "It's happened to me" and your world falls apart. The nightmare of coping with the sexual abuse of your child begins. What do you do in the days to come? What do you say to your child? How will it affect your child's life? Will she or he ever get over it? Will your child grow up to be an offender? Will it happen again?

This book is a parent's guide for talking about sexual abuse with a child who has been victimized. It will help you find your role in your child's recovery.

This book is not intended to help you find out more about what happened to your child; it is not meant to help you be a "fact finder" or detective. Nor will it teach you to be your child's professional counselor. You are too close. Neither role is best for a parent.

The role of a parent is different from that of any other person involved. You are there when the nightmares happen. You provide the limits on sexually aggressive or manipulative behavior. You provide your child's day-to-day sense of security, and you can encourage your child's growth and recovery within that security. You are the most important person in your child's life. There is no one more essential to your child's recovery from the trauma of sexual abuse.

This book will help you and your child to

weather the trauma, pain and losses
heal as your child grows
protect your child from re-abuse, and
grow beyond the hurt

Each situation of abuse is different, each child is different, and every family is different, but some of the difficulties faced after the disclosure of abuse are the same. Parents quickly discover that there is usually little help available beyond basic information about sexual abuse. Parents are often left out of legal, medical, and therapeutic procedures. Up until now, parents have been on their own.

You are not alone. This book has been created from the experiences of parents who have been through what you are going through. Using this workbook will help your child to feel better and behave better. She or he will feel stronger, safer, braver, more lovable, worthwhile, and competent.

Nothing can change the fact that sexual abuse has happened to your child. Your task now is to find a way to live with it—in the best possible way you can.

Together, you and your child can make this happen.

NOTES ON USING THIS BOOK

One of the hardest things for parents is knowing what to say to their child about the sexual abuse. Because of this, the pages of this guide are arranged so that parents' information is on the left-hand page, and examples of what might be said to a child, or activities for parent and child, are on the right-hand page. If your child happens to come sit down next to you while you are reading, there are things you can immediately share. Not all of the examples will fit your child. They are offered as general guidelines.

This guide is not intended to be read front to back. It is arranged so that parents can pick and choose what is most helpful. It is not a substitute for therapy sessions for your child, especially if your child was abused by a family member or someone else very important to her or him.

Since both boys and girls are abused sexually, we have chosen to use she/he when referring to child victims, except in places where it becomes too awkward. In those cases we have chosen to say either he or she. Since the majority of offenders are male, we have chosen for the sake of simplicity to use he when referring to abusers. We do not mean by this that there are no female abusers. In places that refer to the abuser, sometimes we substitute "Xxxxx" with the intention that the parent fill in the name of the abuser if possible.

Most of the quotes contained in the book are not individual stories but composites, or they are from parents who have expressed themselves in public places, in the media, or at conferences. There are also quotes from parents and children who have given permission for their use.

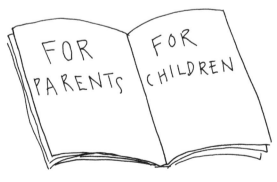

ACKNOWLEDGMENTS

No book is written by the authors alone. Many people helped us at different stages of this project; we owe a debt of gratitude to them. Janet Sherman, Branch Executive of Children's Home Society of Washington, Southwest Branch, believed in this project from the beginning, and played a major role in seeing it through. Pat Beckett of Children's Home Society's Child Sexual Abuse Treatment Program provided many hours of support and contributed her expertise to the workbook. Helen Sullivan offered her comments early on, and was a reader of the final copy, as were Bob Mow and Louise Anderson, all treatment staff of Children's Home Society, Southwest Branch.

There were many others who provided us help through interviews or critical readings of the manuscript, including Margaret Eastman of the Children's Program who encouraged this workbook from its start and proved a valuable resource, as did Jan Eaton-Bennette, Diane Ponder and Lorraine Rupert of the Parry Center and Patti Bailey, Incest Treatment Coordinator for Washington County Children's Services Division. Also the following people provided interviews and/or useful feedback: Lucy Berliner, Carmen Stukas, Joan Renner, Jim Peters, Barbara Northcutt, Barbara Ward, Kathryn Day, Pam Lott, Kathy Mare, Karen Bruno and Tess Fegel.

Thanks go also to Robbie, Herb, Ginevra, Elizabeth, Toby and Piper for their support and "deadline patience", as ever.

We would also like to acknowledge all those courageous parents who have shared their struggles with us as they help their children.

C. A.
J. F.

Helping Your Child Recover
from Sexual Abuse

Chapter 1

Right Away . . . *"I believe you"*

"Oh no, it can't be."

"I don't believe it."

"There must be a misunderstanding."

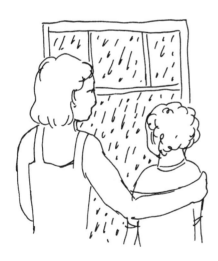

FINDING OUT

Your first task when sexual abuse is disclosed is to separate these natural reactions to overwhelming bad news from disbelief of your child. Your child, or children, need to know that you believe them, and will support them. This feeling that you'll wake up soon and find out it was all a bad dream is called <u>denial</u>. It provides only brief protection from the frustration, misery, horror, and isolation that will follow.

HOW SHOULD YOU ACT?

Children who have someone understanding and supporting them suffer fewer ill effects than do children without help. Your role as a parent is to support your child in recovery, by providing reassurance, safety, and love. You must also make decisions about medical care, legal proceedings, and counseling.

Children need reassurance that they didn't cause your anger, upset, and sadness. Children's belief that they are the cause of everything makes this difficult for them to understand. It is wise to keep your most violent reactions such as "I want to kill the ___, or I feel like my life is over," for other adults. Children can understand your grief if it is not overwhelming.

You can show them you really mean it when you say, "It's okay to cry, be sad or mad."

Now that the secret is out:
    I believe you.
    I'm sorry this happened to you.
    I'm glad I know.
    You will be taken care of.
    I'm not sure what will happen next.

This has happened to other children, your age, younger and older, boys and girls. Nothing <u>about you</u> made it happen.

I will do my best to protect you, now that I know.

You don't need to take care of me.

I know it wasn't your fault.

We will all get over this, just like we recover from illness or an accident, but it may take a long time.

I am upset, but not with you.

I'm angry at the person who did this.

I'm sad. You may see me cry. That's all right. I will be able to take care of you. I'm not mad at you.

Right Away

HOW DO I KNOW MY CHILD IS TELLING THE TRUTH ABOUT THIS?

Children rarely lie about sexual abuse. They are more likely to deny abuse has happened than to make it up. In one study, even the very small number of children thought to be lying about a particular incident had been abused previously and were suffering from flashbacks.

Sometimes children do tell their fantasies as if they had really happened, or insist on the existence of an imaginary friend. But children don't know enough to make up the abusive incidents they describe. They describe in childish words experiences too shocking to be made up. Sometimes the details about time or contact will vary from one telling to another. Children typically remember different parts at different times. They may be trying to stay out of trouble, protecting someone else, or simply responding to stress.

It is easier to believe the abuse didn't occur than to believe that someone, especially someone you know and trust, really does sexually abuse children. It is difficult to believe that adults will use children for their own sexual purposes.

Children may reveal abuse during divorce or custody conflicts. They see the other parent as ready to believe them. Because a few parents do falsely accuse the other of sex abuse in the hope of "automatically" winning custody, the disclosure may be viewed with great suspicion, but it is still most likely accurate.

I know sometimes in the past I haven't believed you. I believe what I have learned about Xxxxx sexually abusing you.

Because your dad (mom) and I are fighting each other right now, some people may be suspicious of what you say. I am not. I know you don't have any reason to lie. I know this is embarrassing and unpleasant. It must have been hard to tell anyone.

I'm proud of your courage and I believe you.

I'm glad you told me.

I'm feeling stunned and I'm not sure what to do. I need to make some phone calls. I believe you; I need some time to think.

What are you most worried about right now?

TAKE CARE OF YOURSELF

You'll be most able to give your child the support she/he needs, no matter how long treatment or legal proceedings take, if you have help yourself. You may blame yourself for not protecting your child. But no parent can be everywhere at all times. Symptoms and signs can be hard to see—though they may seem obvious after the abuse is disclosed. Very few children come right out and tell their parents.

You may face some unpleasant but not unusual surprises:

- You may be isolated because people believe the offender instead of you and your child.
- Your child may be angry with you for your inability to protect him/her. Children often think adults know everything.
- You may learn that your other children were also abused.
- You may remember sexual abuse in your own childhood.
- The abuser will deny the abuse or blame you and your child.

Find people to support you who understand that you did not "allow" your child to be abused. Who would you call on if a child were gravely ill, or you had a fire? Ask them for help now. Don't wait until you are at the end of your energy and patience. Ask for what you need: babysitting, listening, praise for your parenting, to come over and have coffee with you. If you don't have a friend to help, look for a rape crisis or mental health hotline, a social service agency, a women's center, YWCA, YMCA or a member of the clergy knowledgeable and trained about sexual abuse. Keep looking until you find someone. If you remember abuse in your own childhood, you may want to find an adult survivors' group to join.

It isn't your fault or our fault this happened. Usually no one takes advantage of us even if we break a rule.

It took someone willing to act in a way that is wrong to make this happen.

You and I may have different feelings about this. I may be sad when you are mad.

You may have forgotten for a while and I'll still be worrying. It's okay for us to feel differently.

This has happened in other families. We aren't alone. Other families have survived.

I'm sorry it happened. It wasn't your fault.

Others are here to help us. The doctor, police officer, your counselor, my friend, and grandma are helping us. Who else can you think of?

I'm sorry I didn't realize what was happening to you. Now I see what you were trying to tell me.

A FEW "DON'TS"

Don't restrict your child's play or other activities any more than you must for your own peace of mind. If you keep your child from bicycle riding or playing outside, she/he may see this as punishment.

If your child wants to cling to you for a few days, don't be afraid to let her/him. She/he may need lots of reassurance and help feeling safe again.

Don't let your desire to make sense of what has happened lead you into probing questions about details of the abuse. Sometimes children can't give them, or will only tell the story once, or will feel your pressure and reaction and decide to "forget" the whole thing.

Don't ask why they didn't say "no" or tell sooner, because that can increase their feelings of guilt.

Don't be in a hurry to provide reassurances about sexuality such as "Sex in marriage isn't like that." Children can't make sense of that statement. Don't link what happened to them with things you label "bad" (such as pornography).

Don't make any promises about what will happen to the offender, or promise that the child will never have to see the offender again. It may not be true. Your child needs to trust your word. It is better to say you don't know.

Don't urge the child to just try to forget it.

Don't let the child believe she or he caused the misery or pain in the family because she/he told about what was happening.

I know you just wanted the sexual abuse to stop. You didn't want to get anyone in trouble. Telling was the only way it was going to stop. It's not your fault he needs help with his problem.

I know you can take care of yourself, but for a few days I need to see you close by. Please check in every once in a while for me.

It's not being a baby to need a light on, or to need me beside you until you fall asleep. When you feel safe again will be soon enough to give that up.

All this sexual abuse stuff is pretty confusing isn't it? Adults should know better. Adults are confused about sex too. But they should know better.

I don't know what will happen to Xxxxx. He might go see a counselor. He might not be forced to do anything. You didn't make him feel any worse than he did already. If he ever gets healthy, he will be glad you told.

He had a problem. His problem didn't begin with you. Now, he has a chance to get some help.

It's okay to want him to be punished.

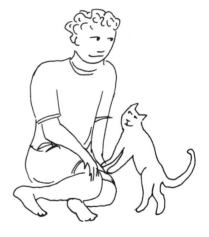

Right Away

9

MEDICAL CARE?

Your child needs an M.D. with special training in responding to child victims of sexual assault. Your community mental health, public health, or rape crisis center should be able to help you locate the medical facility where pediatricians trained to provide care for sexual abuse victims will examine your child.

The doctor should:

- make your child feel comfortable
- establish discussion about the sexual abuse
- reassure the child that telling was a good idea and she/he is not to blame

The doctor should document:

- the emotional state of the child
- what parts of the child's body were involved, using the child's words
- what form the sexual contact took

He or she should also:

- document and treat any physical injury
- test for/prevent infections
- test for pregnancy/provide interventions
- reassure the child she/he is all right from head to toe

If an incident just occurred and you must rush to an emergency room:

- take a change of clothes for your child
- don't bathe the child before going
- call ahead so that the emergency room knows you are coming—sometimes that will lessen the wait

We are going to go see the doctor. She/he will probably ask you quite a few questions so that she knows just what happened.

The doctor will be gentle. If you are afraid, tell the doctor or nurse.

She will examine your body to be sure everything is okay. The doctor will need to examine all of your body, including those parts involved in the abuse, your private parts [or genitals]. This touching and looking is for your health and is okay.

You can ask her/him questions you are embarrassed to ask me.

Is there anything you want me to ask her/him for you?

I know this might be embarrassing or scary or make you nervous. It won't last forever. It is not the same as the abuse.

I'll stay with you.

REPORT TO THE POLICE?

Getting medical attention may result in a report to the agency responsible for protecting children from child abuse, or to the police. Medical personnel are required to report suspected sexual abuse. Ask if the clinic is planning to report.

If they are not, you must make the decision.

REASONS TO REPORT

- Your child may be reassured by contact with the police.
- Sexual abuse is a crime. The only way someone can be stopped is through legal intervention.
- The police can investigate and decide if there is enough evidence to establish a crime.
- Children's sense of justice may be satisfied by legal action.
- Few cases actually go to trial. They are settled out of court.
- Confronting the offender and/or his family yourself is rarely successful. They almost always deny everything.
- Crime Victim's Compensation (financial assistance for victims of crime) is available only to those who report to the police.

BARRIERS TO REPORTING

- You and your child may fear that the offender will go to jail.
- The police may be seen as the enemy in your community.
- You may believe: "We can take care of this ourselves."
- You're afraid you might be accusing an "innocent" man.
- You're afraid of what your child will have to go through.
- You don't want to betray another family, or risk retaliation.

The police are coming to talk to you, not to take you to jail. You haven't broken the law. You will not go to jail.

They will ask you many questions.

Has a police officer ever come to your school to talk to you about safety?

Talking to the police is probably <u>not</u> going to be the way it looks on television. They may not wear a uniform. I don't know if the officer will be a man or woman.

If they say anything you don't understand, please ask me, and I'll try to explain it. I may not be right there while they are talking to you, but I'll be close by.

No matter what the police do, I believe what you have told me. They may believe you too, but not be able to do anything.

COUNSELING?

If you are not already in counseling, you may wonder whether your child needs it. When incest occurs, or abuse has continued over a long period, outside help is necessary. What you do as a parent is therapeutic: you listen, you reassure, you provide comfort. But a trained therapist can provide objectivity and distance allowing your child to work through issues too painful for you to tackle together.

If after some time has passed your child:

>   still won't talk about the abuse,
>
>   is no less fearful,
>
>   seems to be holding something back
>
>   still has not returned to day to day routine, or
>
>   is beginning to act out the abuse with other children

then help is needed. A good counselor can create a safe atmosphere where a child can feel free to show hidden fears and anger.

If you have any doubt, you can consult with a counselor yourself. The best help for you and your child will involve you in your child's treatment. The counselor will recognize you as an essential element of your child's recovery. You can't be included in every session, but you certainly should understand the general direction of what is happening. You need to understand what the counselor is saying and feel that you can ask questions.

If you or your child don't trust or find helpful a particular counselor, keep looking.

A counselor is a safe adult to explore feelings with. She/he may play with you, tell you stories, or ask you to draw pictures.

She/he can help you feel better.

Today we are going to go talk to Ms. Morris. She is called a counselor. She's another person who may ask a lot of questions (like the police or the doctor) but her reasons are different. She is asking questions to find ways to help you feel better again.

You're not in trouble. This is a person like a doctor, someone who is trained to help other people understand and get over problems having to do with feelings or getting along with other people. This counselor knows how hard it can be to get over sexual abuse all by yourself.

You and she can talk about how you are doing now. She has talked to lots of kids who have been sexually abused and has a lot of ways to help kids with problems like yours that someone else made for them.

She may talk with you or have you play with toys, or draw a picture or tell a story.

She might help you:
    talk to the police or caseworker
    understand what court is all about
    work on problems at school

TAKE A MINUTE

You could take a minute now and review what went through your head as you learned your child had been sexually abused, and what you said to your child. Is there anything you want to change now? It is okay to say, "I was upset when I heard, and I want to be sure you know: I believe you, I am sorry it happened to you, I don't believe it was your fault, and I am going to do the best for you I can."

If you hesitated before acting, your child may not understand why. You may want to explain now.

If you have begun to remember sexual abuse in your own childhood, finding a survivors' group or a counselor knowledgeable about adult survivors may be necessary to separate your needed recovery from your child's recovery process.

I'm sorry I didn't act faster. I didn't know what to do. It didn't have anything to do with doubting you or what you said.

I was confused. It was a total surprise.

I'm sad and angry this happened to you, but I'm not angry at you.

You may see me cry sometimes or be upset, but we will be okay. I will take care of you and of myself.

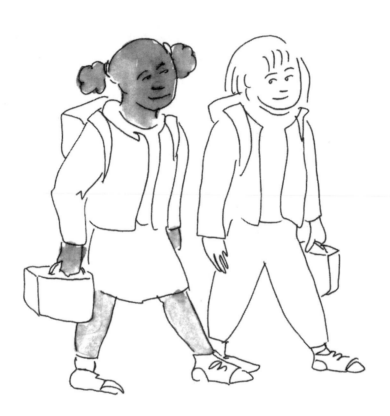

Chapter 2

The Legal System . . . *"They'll be asking a lot of questions"*

"The help we got from everybody was as good as I could have ever imagined. The police officer got right on the floor with Jimmy and let him play with toys during the whole interview. He let Jimmy know what was going to happen next. He introduced the caseworker when she came. Jane (our caseworker) stayed for as long as it took. I really felt she was there to help us. The prosecutor helped him to understand it wasn't his fault. She was so good with him. Jimmy felt much better after going through all these steps."

"Once you report the sexual abuse, you enter the 'twilight zone.' You have no control over what happens. No one returns phone calls. Attorneys try to confuse your child and get her to mix up her story. Things drag on longer than you ever thought possible—it was two years ago when this all started for us. Your child's word is held up to the molester's word, and let me tell you, we all believe children lie and make things up. People play down the impact of the abuse for the sake of the abuser ('He's already suffered enough'). It's a circus."

"I reported the sexual abuse. There was never any doubt in my mind that this guy needed to be held responsible for what he had done. I was expecting to go to court, but they dropped the case. I knew Sheila had been abused, everybody else knew she had been abused, but they said 'insufficient evidence.'"

"The trial was hell, but by God, we got him!"

USING THE LEGAL SYSTEM

It is impossible to predict what will happen for you and your child once the report has been made and you are involved in the legal system. Parents' experiences range from very good to awful. No matter what you expect, there will be surprises.

The legal process can help children feel:
important
cared for
listened to
believed
less burdened
less alone

Children can be relieved to think that someone will tell the offender he was wrong, and help protect them. The chance to speak up about what happened, to be able to say "He did this and I didn't like it", can be a good thing for a child—whether or not the abuser is convicted.

There can be positive outcomes for you, too:

- You can use the legal system to help your child feel safe, to let your child know that you believe her or him and are doing everything you can. (Many adults, when recalling their own abuse as children, express intense anger and feelings of betrayal toward a person they had told about the abuse, but who they felt had done nothing about it.) You may use the legal system to protect your child from future unsupervised contacts with the offender.

- Using the power of the legal system is also a way to try to keep other children safe. Experts say most offenders abuse many more kids than those they have been caught molesting. One study found that some child molesters average 75 victims.

- The legal system is the only way you can hold the offender accountable for what he has done, or help him get treatment. Offenders do not stay in treatment without the force of the legal system behind them.

The Legal System
20

I have to tell some special people what happened to you.

Your teacher had to tell the authorities, because it is her job to help protect children.

You may be wondering why you have to tell so many different people what happened to you. It's because there are laws about sexual abuse that are meant to stop people like Xxxxx from doing what he did. There are people whose job it is to help protect you from more abuse.

Laws are like rules, only more serious. What Xxxxx did to you was against the law.

People ask a lot of questions and try to collect all the facts. Lots of girls and boys have had this happen to them too. They told what happened to them to all these people too. You are the only one who can tell what happened to you.

It's out of our hands now. The people whose job it is to decide what to do about Xxxxx are making the decisions now.

There are other people who are making decisions about our family now.

You may feel afraid that Xxxxx will do what he threatened because you told. He said or did those things to scare and trick you. You are safe now. I will protect you.

He made all this happen, not you. When adults break the law, they deserve to be punished by other adults.

It's good that you told.

It's not to punish Xxxxx, but to stop him from hurting other children. He needs help to stop. What Xxxxx did was wrong. He needs to learn that, and this is the only way I know how to get that to happen.

WHAT MAKES THE PROCESS HARD

Not knowing how the system works or what to expect—The legal system was not designed with the needs of children in mind. The basis of our criminal justice system is the protection of the rights of the accused. The rights of the child victim are far less defined than the rights of the accused abuser. The system does not work well for child sexual abuse victims. However, across the country, efforts are being made to improve the legal system's response to child abuse by:

- Giving child abuse cases priority in court schedules

- Reducing the number of times the child has to tell her/his story to justice system personnel and the total number of interviews (one way is recording or videotaping the child's first interview with a professional)

- Using live two-way, closed-circuit television for grand jury appearances and sometimes for the trial itself (at present, children are required to face the accused offender, which is hard for most children

- Tailoring the length of the testimony to the age of the child and excluding spectators from the courtroom (even little kids must sometimes testify for hours)

- Keeping the same prosecutor throughout

- Improving the background and expertise of judges and other legal professionals on the topic of child abuse

- Training attorneys and judges to interview in a manner appropriate for the child's development

Having no control over what happens—Phone calls may not be returned, and you may not be notified when critical things happen, such as the offender being let out on bail. Decisions are made without your knowledge. If you are feeling bad, or out of control and helpless, it's no wonder. Remember that your child is a witness for the state. The prosecutor is not your personal attorney, but rather the state's attorney, because child abuse is a crime against the state.

You don't have to protect me from the story.

I will not leave you.

I still care about you.

I'm not sorry that other people know.

I'm not mad at you.

I'm sorry that others seem mad at you.

You may be worried about Xxxxx. You may think "I've made him feel bad." Remember Xxxxx started this, not you, and he should have known better.

Sometimes people need to feel bad before they are willing to get help.

I don't know what will happen to Xxxxx:
    maybe jail
    maybe he will get some help
    maybe not very much at all will happen

I don't know why he did it. He has a problem.

You can still love someone but hate what they did to you.

Not always being able to be with your child—Many times parents are asked to wait while the child is being questioned. Being left out of the various proceedings can make you feel that you are not very important to the process, or to your child. People can seem rude and curt, as though they have no time for you. You're "just a parent," and besides, you may "contaminate" the proceedings. Many interviewers prefer the parent not be present because they feel the interview will go better and they will get better information if you are not there. The child may be reluctant to tell details, wanting to spare you from them. Sometimes parents cannot contain their emotional distress at what they hear, or may pressure the child unnecessarily to get them to tell.

A good interviewer will take the time to make sure your child is comfortable without you, perhaps by seeing you both together for a while and then showing your child where you will be during the interview. It should be clear that the parent is available, if necessary. Other interviewers think it is better not to interview children alone, especially younger children. Talk this out with the caseworker, police officer, or attorney before the interview, if you are able.

The timing—The legal process goes on at its own pace, regardless of the need of the child to heal. The emotional wounds are reopened by the various proceedings, perhaps over a period of a year or two, unpredictably interrupting the recovery process. Your court date may be delayed over and over again. You have no control over this process.

It's hard for most children to talk about sexual abuse. To have to talk about it many times (for example to the police, the child protective caseworker, the detective, the prosecutor, the defense attorney, the jury, the judge, the counselor, or even you) can be very hard for a child. Some stop talking. An insensitive or untrained interviewer can add to the child's sense of guilt and make him feel that people blame or disbelieve him.

Kids may begin to regret the telling. They do not feel "safe" when they don't know when they might have to go talk to someone again.

People in the legal system use a lot of words. There are different words for Xxxxx, different words for sexual abuse. You may be hearing these words and wonder what they mean. If you hear a word you want to understand better, ask me. I'll try to explain.

Mr. Evans feels it is better for you to talk to him alone because sometimes it's easier for kids to talk when their parents aren't around.

I know I said this morning that you wouldn't have to go to the prosecutor's office anymore, but I got a call today from him and he says if we come in one more time, probably it will be the last. I'm sorry about this. I know how tired you are of all the questions. Afterwards, lets go to the park and we can buy some popcorn as a reward for getting through it.

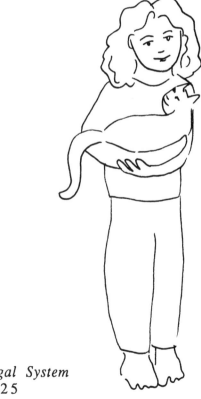

The Legal System
25

THE INTERVIEWS—WHAT TO DO

Find an advocate for yourself who is sympathetic and familiar with child sexual abuse cases. Call your local rape crisis center, counselor, caseworker, prosecutor, or police officer and ask. There may be a Victim/Witness Program available that keeps the victim notified of the status of the case (court dates, etc.), helps the victim negotiate the legal system, follows up if there is a conviction, and assists in getting possible compensation. There may be a Guardian Ad Litem Program available to provide your child with an advocate. Prosecutors are too overworked to be your best ally. You need another. You have the right to have an advocate with you at all times.

Don't be afraid to make a phone call to ask questions about what will happen next, or how a decision was made. You have the right to information about your child's case.

Don't think it's you. The legal system is very complex. If you don't understand, don't be surprised. Even its own employees have difficulties describing how the system works—in every county and state it is different, and it changes all the time.

Prepare your child for the interviews. Be calm and reassuring, or matter-of-fact. Don't coach the child about what to say. It's important for the story to come out in your child's words, in your child's own time. The legal system has little awareness of your child's physical needs, so take food, tissues, crayons, a favorite book or toy, and ask where the bathrooms are. Do not talk to the defense attorney (Xxxxx's lawyer) without the prosecutor there with you and the child. Some defense attorneys try to come to your house and say you have to talk. That is not true. Tell him/her to contact the prosecutor.

Have rewards for you and your child even if something doesn't happen, because it's hard to get prepared for an interview or hearing and then have it delayed. Make the rewards independent of the success or failure of the interview or the case in general. Make it a reward for "getting through the interview," rather than a reward for "how well you told your story." Have backup activities planned. For instance, go to the park or a shopping mall, or go and watch the airplanes take off and land.

You will be talking to Mr. Smith today about what has been happening.

We are going to the courthouse today to talk to Ms. Jones about the sexual abuse.

You will be telling what happened to you. I know it's hard to talk about.

I'm going to be right outside here. Don't worry about me.

Are you uncomfortable going to talk with Mrs. Black? What are you most worried about? We can talk about it.

Xxxxx will have his attorney too. You don't ever need to talk to Xxxxx's attorney alone, even if he asks you to.

I don't know what is going to happen next, but I do know I'll be right here trying to do my best to help us get through this.

Let's go for ice cream as a reward for getting through a hard day.

Let's go to the park after this to feed the ducks.

In the best of all possible worlds, what would you like to happen now? When things get hard, imagine:
>   seeing a sunset
>   smelling fresh air
>   feeling the cool lake water on a hot summer day

It is a good picture to keep in your head.

A trip to the courtroom

More and more often, child sexual abuse cases never get to the courtroom. Many cases are plea bargained. This is a legal process in which the offender pleads guilty, usually to a lesser charge. (Studies show that in some areas of the country, only 2% of children ever appear in court. On the average, only 31% of the non-family and 23% of the family cases involve court action.)

If the prosecuting attorney, victim advocate, counselor, or caseworker hasn't already done so, take your child to the courtroom and show her/him around, or ask to be taken there together. Let her/him sit in the witness chair and the judge's and jury's chairs. Tell her/him where you will be sitting and where the judge will be sitting. Let the child know that the judge is human—probably has children— and wears the funny robe so people will know who he or she is. Tell your child where Xxxxx will be sitting. (This is a way to present the fact that Xxxxx will be there.)

Children facing a court trial worry about:
- Seeing the abuser again
- All those people who ask questions
- Not wanting to go; wanting it to be over
- Being scared (maybe Xxxxx will make good on his threats)
- Embarrassment (it is hard to talk about sexual abuse in front of people)
- People doing all this because she/he told about the abuse.
- What to say if they don't know the answer
- Wondering where mom will be

If you are also a witness, you will not be allowed in the courtroom when your child is testifying. There are some good sides to this. It just may be easier on the child not to have you there. But there is no way your child should ever be in the courtroom without an ally present in addition to the prosecutor. Make sure an advocate, your best friend, a relative—someone the child trusts—is there too. In fact, this person can stay with the child at all times.

You know we are going to go to the courtroom this morning and you will be asked to talk about what happened. Everybody gets nervous going to court. That's normal. To stay calm, let's breath deeply, think about a favorite place, or draw a picture.

I know it's been hard. But I'll be there with you.

I may not be able to be with you all the time today, but that is why Joni from the advocate program is here. She understands what it's like for kids. She can be there for you when I'm not.

What about court worries you most? The courtroom is a safe place.

It's okay to cry in the courtroom. Lots of people have. Everyone understands, and it's good to show just how you really feel. You don't have to pretend not to care.

You are not responsible for Xxxxx's problems. Xxxxx needs to get help. That's why he is there. He needs to figure out that what he did wasn't right.

It's good that you are talking about the abuse. No matter what, you are okay. A lot of people care about you and want to do what needs to be done.

Assuming that your child is judged competent as a witness, she/he will probably be brought before the person who abused her/him and required to talk about what happened. Many are too young, or too traumatized to be considered competent (a legal judgment only). Some children are simply not old enough to be able to talk about the abuse in a convincing way.

Kids know that the abuser is saying "I didn't do it" or "She made me do it" or "It was no big deal." They begin to doubt their own memories. We teach kids to tell the truth. They may be shocked by the offender's lies.

Some kids do okay with facing the offender in court. Others are very afraid, and sometimes even recant (take back their story or statement) in order to avoid court and the offender.

Bring all the supportive people you can to the courtroom, if that is okay with your child. If someone is not in total support—or even hints disbelief—don't bring that person.

I'm not sure what will happen next. I think we may have to wait all morning or come back again tomorrow. Next I think they will ask questions of your counselor.

Look at me, not at Xxxxx or at the prosecuting attorney. He may try to glare at you, so you can just look at me or your support person. Ignore Xxxxx's tricks (of staring, sighing, gasping, whispering). He's trying to make you nervous. He may have threatened you with harm, but he was just trying to scare you and trick you.

He can't yell at you, or hurt you. He can't yell that you are lying. The jury would think he is a real jerk. His attorney will tell him not to do that.

Here is a ring (rabbit's foot, picture) that you can keep in your pocket. It means I love you. When I can't be with you, think of the ring and it will help you be brave.

What are you most afraid of? What is hardest for you? Here is a rock crystal for you to wear under your shirt. I have a matching one that I'm wearing on my necktie. They mean we care about each other, even when we are apart.

If they ask you something you don't understand, it's okay to say "I don't understand." Don't say "I don't know." Just say you don't understand the question, and they will explain it or ask it another way.

Notebook—Keep a notebook with your child that is a record of these days and what happens. At the end of the day, for example, ask the child what was hardest, or what she/he liked the best. Record those in your shared notebook. It is a way to "debrief" and let out some of the stress of the day. Write unsent letters (to the judge, prosecutor, defense attorney, caseworker) about how you would have liked to see things go today. Write all the things you would like to say to this person in your letter, then don't send it. Put it in your notebook.

The system can't make it right or fix it

Most of us expect a crime as serious as child sexual abuse to be recognized and punished by the power of the law—that reporting it means justice will be done. But it is never that simple.

You might be expecting that the legal system can "fix" what happened. It can't. The legal system cannot make what happened right again. Even if you are lucky, all goes well, and you feel justice has been done, justice alone will not bring recovery to your child.

It is best to enter the legal system without expectations and with the attitude that it is a drama, a complicated process, but one that is not essential to your child's recovery. The more you expect justice, the harder the experience is likely to be.

Try to keep in mind what your objective is: the well-being of your child. Don't lose yourself to the legal system. The outcome is not essential to your child's well-being. It can be only one step in your child's recovery process.

No matter how painful it is for you to work your way through the jungle that the legal system can be, remember this fact: day after day, counselors who talk with adults who were molested as children hear one thing, "My parents didn't do anything." This feeling can cause untold repercussions for the child, lasting for years. Your child will never say that.

Doing everything you can to make the statement that abusing your child won't be tolerated (no matter how difficult) is essential to your child's well-being.

Reduce the offender's power:

"Let's draw a picture of Xxxxx. What would you like to do with it?
     Scribble him out?
     See how he looks sitting on a pig?
     Tape it on the wall?
     Tear it up and throw it away?

Let's talk about our feelings. How did you feel when the defense attorney confused you about the time? That's his job, to tell Xxxxx's story, and Xxxxx has changed his story because he doesn't know any better. He thinks he can get away with lying. The defense attorney knows you are telling the truth, but he can't act that way because he is working for Xxxxx.

CELEBRATE when it's over. No matter the outcome, conviction or not. Tell the child it is over: "We did our best to see that Xxxxx gets help. That's the best we can do." Or that you and the child did your best, worked hard, put in a lot of time, and now it's over. Celebrate the job well done. Tell your child: "You don't have to worry about him. This celebration is for you. It's time for you to feel better now." You could have a party and invite the prosecutor, a caseworker, or kids from a therapy group. Have a cake, give cards or presents.

How do you present the outcome of the legal process to the child?

It is important to continue to separate the legal action from what you and the child know to be the reality of events. Just because child protective services, or the detective, or the court makes their investigation and decides that there is not enough evidence to confirm the abuse <u>does not mean that the abuse did not occur, or that your child does not need help, or that the offender is not an abusive person</u>. Don't leave it to the legal system to decide whether your child has been abused, when you already know she/he was. You might ask the prosecutor to write a letter to the child telling him he was believed, he did a good job, and he doesn't need to come to court again.

Kids under the age of five are unlikely to ask the outcome, and don't particularly understand the concept anyway. Follow the young child's lead. If she/he doesn't ask, you don't need to tell. Don't share your own frustration and feelings of powerlessness with your child; find another sounding board.

When the legal process ends, expect to feel let down, or to have a period of depression, even if it has been a positive experience. It happens to most parents.

You are looking for a sense of relief, since it's over finally; but it doesn't come. You've had to put your previous emotions on hold to get by, perhaps without realizing it. But the problem isn't fixed, and your child is not "back to normal."

Remember:

- Even if the case is dropped, you have done your best in trying to prevent further abuse and to hold the offender responsible for what he did. <u>That is a major accomplishment</u>.

- Offenders go on to repeat their crime if they don't get help. There is only one thing that keeps most offenders in treatment: legal pressure.

- You have other options, such as bringing a civil suit against the offender. One family brought suit against another family, and their home owner's insurance paid damages.

The Legal System
34

Just because they didn't find Xxxxx guilty, that doesn't mean they didn't believe you. They do know that the abuse really happened. But they have to follow the court's rules.

Xxxxx was not found guilty in court, but that doesn't mean he didn't really do the sexual abuse. It just means the evidence wasn't enough to prove him guilty under the court's rules. It takes lots of proof.

The judge believes you—he just has to follow the court's rules, and there has to be lots of proof.

You may be wondering how someone can do something wrong or against the law and not be punished. It doesn't make sense to me either.

It's over. No more going to the courthouse. Now it's time to concentrate on you. It's time for you to feel better.

It doesn't matter what the court process did. What matters is that you did what you needed to do.

The judge decides what to do now.

You are safe. You have been very brave.

Now it is time to take care of you.

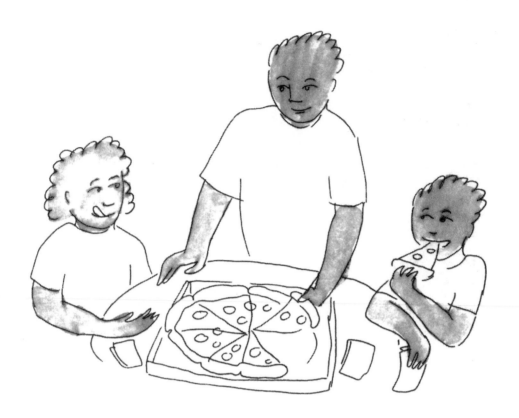

Chapter 3

Family and Friends' Responses . . . *"She cares, but she doesn't understand"*

"I know how hard this is, because I've been there."

"We all knew about Uncle Joe. Didn't you know better than to leave him with the kids?"

"Gosh, I never leave my children with people like that."

"Your son was abused by a woman? How can that be sexual abuse?"

SOME WILL HELP

Sometimes people are very sympathetic, listen and cry with you, and help you plan what to do. You may be relieved that so many of the people in your life have come forward. Sometimes people blame you for what happened to your child. You may be feeling angry and isolated.

When your child is aware that others "know," she/he may need help understanding what their reactions mean. Children deserve the positive comfort and security that comes from friends and family. Rejection by people who know about the abuse is extra hard on kids. So is any hint that loved ones blame your child, or don't believe her/him. This adds to the guilt, shame, and feelings of being bad, different, or unlovable that abused children may have.

It is too big a job for you to change people's attitudes, but you can counter any blaming messages from family or friends your child hears. Help your daughter or son understand what causes people to say such things and that the cause is not her/him.

Remember what Aunt Sylvie says? You'll always be the "apple of her eye." She means it.

Mrs. Jones and her daughter Emily are coming over today. She said she wants to visit us because she knows how hard recovering from sexual abuse can be.

I know you didn't want Uncle Fred to know, but someone told him. You don't have to do or say anything about that.

You can decide who to tell. You don't have to tell everyone.

Grandma still loves you, but is sorting out her feelings. She is upset and confused about what Xxxxx did.

WHAT THEY WILL SAY

Here are some typical responses. You may find your own experience in these voices, and so may your child.

"A neighbor of ours, a friend I thought, told all the other neighbors. They all stopped letting their kids come to play. My kids were miserable."

For this parent, privacy was invaded; for the kids, there are new feelings of rejection to deal with.

Why didn't she say no? Didn't she get the school program about touching? Didn't you tell her to say no?"

In trying to understand how the offender could do what he did, people will deny the seriousness of the impact on your child, or will want very much to find someone or something else to blame (you, your child, the offender's wife, his own past abuse suffered) anything but him.

"I can't believe Fred would do anything like that. Are you sure little Susan hasn't heard that from someone else? Some of those dirty kids from the apartments near the park?"

People are shocked beyond understanding at the thought of what some people are doing to children. One of the hardest things about sexual abuse is the secrecy, denial, and blaming that surrounds it. Everybody wants to forget it, everybody wants you to stop making such a big deal of it— "it wasn't that bad."

"I think you ought to try to forget about it now. You know talking about it only makes it worse for your child. If you don't talk about it to him, he'll forget it."

Some people still think that not talking about abuse makes it go away. They may even go so far as to tell this to your child.

"But really, didn't you know it was going on in your house? How can you not know something like that. Why didn't you stop him?"

Some people may blame you for not protecting your child from the abuse.

Yes, Johnny, Aunt Sue cares about you. She just doesn't understand. Sometimes people say dumb or wrong things because they don't know any better.

You know, a lot of people forget that you might have said no but Xxxxx didn't listen. They forget that it shouldn't be up to children to stop adults.

She doesn't understand what sexual abuse is and how the child is not to blame. It doesn't mean she doesn't love you anymore.

We know a lot now about sexual abuse that other people don't, like some people know a lot about boating or stamp collecting. That's why some of your friends don't come over here now. They don't understand. I know that it's hard. But there is some pain we can't make right again.

Let's practice what you can say if someone says something you don't like:

"I'm doing fine."

"I don't want to talk about it, thank you."

"He's got the problem, not me."

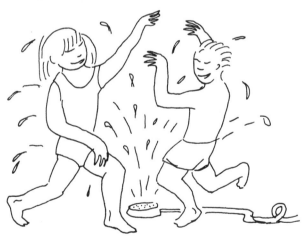

Family and Friends' Responses

41

TAKING SIDES

Brothers and sisters can be a great support, or they can be resentful. All their anger may be directed at the child who told. If this is the case, it is important to see that at least the parts of this workbook about blaming and fault are gone over with the brothers or sisters. The rest of the workbook could help them too. It might also be that a brother or sister who knew about the abuse and didn't tell is feeling confused and guilty and needs to know that there is nothing that he or she could have done.

Sometimes whole organizations take sides as well. For example, it is not unheard of for a school's entire population of parents, students, and teachers to sign a petition saying how outstanding the principal is (the one you have accused of sexual abuse, who has probably molested kids at that school for years). Support may continue even after he has been convicted—sometimes it grows stronger.

"You'll ruin the career of a good man. He's loved kids all his life."

PROBLEMS BETWEEN PARTNERS

Under the stress of disclosed sexual abuse, problems between partners tend to surface. The added strains push both of you to the end of your rope. Its normal to react this way under pressure. You and your partner may be having very different reactions. For instance, a husband may hold in his anger, not talk, and want to be alone. A wife may respond by talking continually to whoever will listen and seeking out support agencies in the community. Or one partner may seek sexual contact for comfort and closeness during this time, while the other is feeling repulsed by the idea of sex in general.

If your partner's reaction is different from yours, you may think that he or she cares less about what happened. That usually isn't true. It's more likely that the two of you have very different ways of coping with stress. Try to remember that when neighbors say things like:

"Gee, Lois, I don't understand how Jeff can be so calm. I know if our daughter had been abused, Herb would have just gone out and killed the guy."

You know, when you hear the upset in people's voices, you may be sorry you told me.

You may be angry about everything that has happened since I found out. I don't blame you—it's been hard for you.

You may feel upset because we don't go to visit Grandpa's anymore. You said you think he might be lonely. Well, we can't visit Grandpa anymore until he is well. He isn't well yet.

You're right, it's not your fault. I just don't want to worry while you are there. Grandma is not able to protect you; she is still upset because of what Grandpa did.

I'm sorry you can't ride the horse—that was fun and now you can't do it anymore. But I can't keep you safe there as long as your cousins don't get help.

You are better now, but it takes older people longer.

I know your brothers and sisters have been acting angry with you. It is really tough to be blamed for someone else's problems.

It's frightening to hear people talk about killing someone, isn't it? They don't mean it. It's their way of trying not to be scared.

ISOLATION

Being blamed by the people you care about for something the offender did is a shock and a betrayal. It can make you feel very alone and isolated. It can cause you to doubt the seriousness of the abuse, or to doubt yourself.

During this process, you may even recall your own abuse or begin to remember more about it. This often happens. It's likely to make you unable to respond to your child in the way she/he needs right now, because it takes everything you have to deal with your own feelings. For instance, you may know in your mind that it isn't your child's fault, but you may hear yourself saying such things as "Why didn't you tell me before" or Don't you know better than to do that?" Perhaps things like that were said to you as a child by a blaming adult, and they are coming to mind repeatedly.

It takes a brave and courageous person to persist through this. It is important that you get support; don't handle this alone.

This is what can help:

Tell your trusted friends what you need from them. They won't know. You may need someone who will listen to what has happened, or someone who will hold you while you cry, or someone who will drive you somewhere, or someone who will tell you that you can get through this, or someone who can tell you how they got through it.

If your child is being teased at school (some kids have words like "slut," "fairy," or "faggot" yelled at them in the hallways), there are some options to try: have a conference with the teacher and/or principal, bring in a speaker about sex abuse prevention, or have a discussion of child abuse. Some parents make the choice of moving or changing schools. It helps to work on your child's own ability to stop the teasing. Help your child to understand that the teasing comes from ignorance.

Sometimes when I'm upset I say things that were said to me as a child. I'm sorry. I'm getting help so I'll stop doing it.

If your friends at school are name calling, they are doing it to pretend they are tough. They are afraid of being sexually abused themselves.

Try telling the teaser to stop. Look him/her in the eye, stand tall, and say in a big voice: "I don't like that. Stop teasing me!"

If the person teasing you seems too big or powerful, try ignoring the teasing.

Handle it like you would other kinds of bullies.

Everybody gets teased, for different things. People who tease you don't know what those things mean to you. They don't know what happened. They're just saying the words.

People say things and call names because of their own fears. It's their problem, not yours.

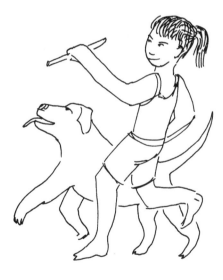

Family and Friends' Responses

FAMILY

If your child is older than seven, decide together just who should be told and how. If your child is younger than seven, it is more your decision. Try to respect your child's wishes about who should know. Children need to find support; they don't know where they stand any more. If you claim that a certain person should not know, think very seriously about the message this gives your child about a connection between sexual abuse and secrecy. You do not want to recreate the secrecy of the abuse by suggesting that it can't be talked about.

Parents and their children have very different concerns about telling. For example, a child may want a favorite grandmother to know, but a parent may fear that grandma will label her as a terrible parent for "letting" this happen. Whatever your decisions about telling, help your child understand that it has nothing to do with blaming her/him.

Non-custodial parents may be a particular problem, using this as an opportunity to challenge custody agreements. If the abuse took place in a non-custodial situation, the fear is the loss of further visits. It may cause an uproar, but keeping a secret from a parent is a dangerous practice.

<u>Do not allow your child to get you to promise to keep the assault totally secret</u>. If you have already promised, tell her/him you made a mistake. You may have to negotiate with your child, but you need an outlet for your own pain and crisis. Vent your feelings about other family members, but don't do it in front of your child.

If your child wants to tell everybody she or he knows, it could be that she/he has been rewarded for telling the story, and wants more reward. In that case, try to reward the child in other ways, and limit the telling. Everyone does not need to know; it's not a secret, but it is private. A child who needs to tell everyone in the world really has another need. It is up to you and/or the child, to decide <u>what</u> to tell. It is not necessary for everyone to hear the details, even if they press you for them.

Who do you think we should tell about this? Who would we tell if you broke a leg? Had your tonsils out?

I know this is embarrassing and sometimes people say thoughtless things, but I need support. Shall we tell Grandma? Aunt Pam? Your father? Your teacher?

Writing Letters—Sent and Unsent

You can write letters, too. One girl, who hadn't seen her father for years, discovered that her sister's counselor had told him. The girl was very angry at this. She felt it was her right to decide who knew about the abuse, since it had happened to her. She wrote a letter to the counselor telling her she was wrong to have done it, that she felt it was her decision, that her dad had not been in her life for nine years and that she was angry that the control had been taken from her as to when he was told. She <u>sent</u> the letter to the counselor and asked her to answer.

The Magic Wand Game

Have the family sit down together. Pass around a Magic Wand that you have made out of wood or paper. Each person gets one wish. It can be anything. No one "corrects" what someone else says. Get into and encourage fantasies and feelings. Make the point to the child that it is not bad to have those feelings. (Acting on them is something else, but the feelings are okay.) Examples: "I wish my father was a toad." You might ask where the toad might live, what it would do, but nothing judgmental.

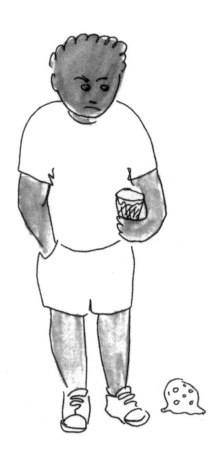

Chapter 4

Children's Reactions and Everyday Life . . . "It's okay to be angry"

"You know, it's okay to be so angry at someone that you wish they were dead. That's a feeling lots of kids and adults have had. Have you ever thought that?"

"You are not alone." "Other kids have felt this way, too and they have also felt better again after some time."

"You may think you'll never feel happy again. It's pretty normal to feel that way after sexual abuse. It's okay. You won't feel sad forever."

WHAT TO EXPECT

Everyday life with your child is probably different from the way it was before the abuse.

Your child may show none of the typical changes in behavior, or may show all of them. Don't feel guilty if a behavior change did not immediately say "sex abuse" to you. It takes time to recognize a pattern, and further time to link behavior changes to sexual abuse rather than to other troubles.

Your reaction to your son's or daughter's everyday behavior can make a difference. What is important now is to help your child express feelings about the abuse and what has happened since. Setting boundaries and limits can show your child that she/he still has a parent who will keep her/his world secure.

There will be hours when children show no symptoms, while playing or off at school. Then, as they remember, the fear or anger comes back. There are children who show no signs or symptoms. Some tend to have stomach aches, headaches, and other aches and pains that are related to anxiety and emotional trauma. Most don't suffer physical traumas of sexual abuse, such as soreness or rashes in the genital/anal area.

Children have their own strengths and abilities. Some children are more fragile than others, and some children seem to be born survivors. Each child is different, each situation of abuse is different, and how the people around the child respond is different. Each plays a part in how a child reacts.

You may be more nervous. You may be frightened but you don't know why. Your tummy may hurt.

You may not enjoy school, or friends the way you used to. You may not like to do things you used to like to do, and you may not be able to think of one thing you like anymore.

What you are going through is normal. It's the way people respond to problems like sexual abuse. It won't last forever.

You deserve help. I want to do my best to help you feel better. It's hard to handle this problem alone.

You know, what has happened is a problem. We've had problems before, and we've worked them out, haven't we? Remember when Grandpa died? Everyone was crying all the time, and we were sad. We missed Grandpa. But now we feel better, don't we? It takes time, but we can take care of this, too.

You found the strength to survive. You got through it.

Remember when we moved here? It was a hard time. We had to do lots of things and meet lots of new people. And you were afraid to make new friends. And it was so scary your first day of school. This is a problem like that was a problem. We did a good job with that one and we'll do a good job with this one.

How do you treat this child now?

Treat your child as normally as you can. Don't throw out all that you know about raising children. Don't stop expecting your child to obey the family rules. Remember you have been raising this child for a long time now and you have a lot of strengths and qualities that have gotten you this far.

Angry Outbursts

Angry outbursts, temper tantrums, or words of hate are common. Let them happen, but make the distinction between feelings and action and set limits on how the anger gets expressed.

Children may be particularly angry with a nonabusing parent. It is safe to be angry at you; it has not been safe to be angry at the offender. The anger may also come from the child's reasoning that if parents are powerful and all knowing they must have "let" the abuse happen. Sometimes kids feel that they have told about the abuse, in so many words, but no one got the message.

Confused Feelings

Children may have many confused feelings about the abuse and what has happened since. Try to discover and listen to those feelings without interrogating or grilling for answers. What the child is feeling is most likely not the same as what you are feeling. Make it safe for the child to express those feelings. Don't be judgmental or try to "correct" the way the child feels, or pressure her/him. Just provide the opportunity. Feelings aren't right or wrong. It is best if those feelings are heard by someone who cares.

Keep your own feelings separate from those of your child. Many younger children feel mainly confusion, and need adult help. They don't need to take on your feelings of distress about the abuse. For instance, many times parents are most concerned about sexuality issues. (Will he be gay? Will she be able to have a normal marital relationship?) For kids, depending on their developmental stage, concerns are more related to control, or body integrity, or feelings of helplessness.

It's okay to explode. It's not okay to hit the family dog or break furniture while you are exploding.

It's okay to be angry, to be sad, to not feel good. You are okay when you feel that way. But it is not okay to kick the cat or break vases because you feel so bad. There are other ways to let those feelings out. You can throw pillows on the floor.

"How are you this morning?"

"Other kids have felt that way, too, when this kind of thing has happened to them." "That makes sense to me." "You have every right to be angry."

Sometimes kids feel: Sad. Mad. Bad. Big mad. Mixed up. Feel like blowing up, like Mount St. Helens. Like it's my fault. It's embarrassing to talk about. Dirty. Like I'm a troublemaker. Like I've let you down. Like Xxxxx won't like me anymore. Lonely because I won't ever see Xxxxx at my house again. The loss of fun things. (We all used to go motor scooting together.)

Art Activity

Provide opportunities for the expression of feelings. You can talk, draw, paint, cut out pictures from a magazine that evoke certain feelings, or use some of the "feelings songs" available on records for preschoolers.

I'm getting out some paper and crayons because I want to draw a picture. Some days it helps me to feel better just to draw. Would you like to draw too?

"I'm coloring a sad picture of how I felt when Xxxxx couldn't baby-sit anymore because he has a touching problem, and over here I'm going to draw a happy picture of how glad I was that you told me about him. Would you like to draw feelings too?" "Can you tell me about your painting?"

Children's Reactions and Everyday Life
53

DREAM WORK

Your child may wake up from nightmares and want the bad dreams to stop. One way to change them is to talk about them, or act them out. Kids could also keep a dream notebook, where they record their dreams right after waking up. They could also draw out a scene or character from their dream. With younger kids it helps to "go with" the dream, helping them by pretending to get the monsters out of the room, for instance. Draw a DREAM HELPER. This is a picture drawn by your child of a powerful, friendly helper who protects children in their dreams. Put it over the bed.

LIMIT TESTING

Biting other children, stealing, kicking the dog, hitting you—your child is being destructive, hostile, and aggressive. Even though this is probably a result of the abuse, don't change the rules you had before the abuse happened. If you are not sure what to do about one of these behaviors, ask yourself how you would have handled it if your child had never been sexually abused, and then handle it like that. It does not help a child when you relax their normal rules and limits; it just makes them feel out of control, and with no one to help them stay in control.

CLINGING

Children who have been abused may seem to want to be your shadow. If she/he wants to be rocked and cuddled frequently, even at very inconvenient times, you should pretty much resign yourself to filling that need. It should decrease with time. If you fight it, the need to cling will probably only increase.

Other kids may just need more chances for physical closeness— cooking together, setting the table together, being together. Older kids may be more withdrawn than clingy, but you still need to be available. Set up times together, like a breakfast time ritual, or an exercise ritual. When an abused child acts in more baby-like ways, let it happen and comfort the child.

I used to have scary dreams too. You know what helped me? I would punch a punching bag. It gave me confidence. If I can't punch him in my dream, like a ghost, then I can outsmart him. What might help you? Or when you see monsters. In your dream, face them and give them a big nose. Make them look funny.

Let's draw a funny monster now.

Being destructive was not okay before, and it is not okay now.

You don't get to kick the dog when you are feeling this way. Don't take it out on the dog. Come tell me what you were thinking when you decided to do that.

Don't hit me. It's not okay to hit people in this house. That is a family rule. I know you are very mad at me. I don't blame you for being mad, you have the right to be mad. Can you tell me about it? Or tear up these newspapers instead?

You may have "flashbacks" or reruns in your head of what happened when you were abused. That is normal; it happens. It might be scary for you, but it is not real, even though it feels real.

Okay, family, it's "Snuggle Time"!

Here is a stuffed animal for you to hug and sleep with.

This puppet has long arms and legs that wrap around you in a nice way.

WHAT ABOUT SLEEPING IN THE SAME BED?

Children may try to take care of adults by offering to sleep with them. You won't know why your child wants to sleep in your bed unless you ask. If the child wants to comfort you by sleeping in your bed, you need to tell her/him that you may be sad, or lonely, but that you are all right. You can thank your child for being thoughtful.

If she/he needs comforting, and is young, you need to make a decision about how wise sleeping in the same bed is. It may start a habit that is hard to change. Maybe it would be better for you to go to her/his bed or room and sit with the child for a while, until she/he can sleep.

Fears and Phobias

You may have already found that a night light and stuffed animals can be of some comfort. Kids tend to make up their own rituals. They rig up bells that will ring if anyone comes in their bedroom door; they ask you to check them in bed every hour; they may coach a doll about being brave every night at bedtime.

Kids set up rituals to diminish their fears, and they do seem to work. If the fears don't decrease after a few months, or if the need for rituals seems excessive, be sure the child sees a professional who can help.

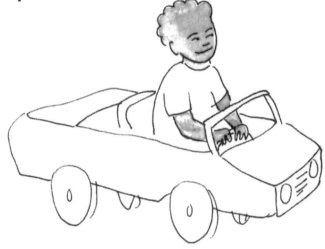

Children's Reactions and Everyday Life

You don't need to take care of me this way. I'm feeling lonely, but I'm all right.

You can crawl into bed with us in an emergency (like when there is thunder and lightening you crawl into our bed till the storm is quiet), but I'd like for you to go to sleep in your own bed as soon as you can.

If you need, I will stay with you while you fall asleep.

I know you want me to lie down with you until you are asleep. I can do that for just a while. We both need our own beds and our own privacy.

What would make you feel safer? I will put a light in the hall for you. Any other ideas?

I will do my part in the bedtime routine you have made up to feel safe:

We can sing "Whistle a Happy Tune" together,

then I tuck you in tightly,

then I turn on the light in the hall.

Emotional Swings

Some kids are fine, then they are crying, angry, demanding, or unable to handle change. Some kids are withdrawn, wanting to be alone. Then they act like their old selves again. Some are passive, aggressive, depressed, sarcastic, or have tantrums and angry outbursts.

These mood swings are part of getting better. They should decrease over time. You might keep a notebook with the date and any symptoms, such as angry outbursts or tantrums. You might find that your child's behavior is related to how you are feeling, too. Sometimes kids react when they see parents being overwhelmed, and they do it in an effort to get the parent back on track. In that case, you could learn to anticipate tantrums.

Let your child know you will comfort her/him when the sad feelings come up; that you will help them to release the anger and to express other feelings. It often helps to release feelings physically, for example, by slamming doors or throwing a ball hard against an outside wall.

Acting Out

Many kids who have been abused will be sexually aggressive toward another, usually younger, child. Don't be afraid to react. Your child is really looking for a reaction. Your response helps your child to understand the meaning of the sexual abuse. When you respond by stopping the behavior, saying that it is not okay to make other people do things like that, or that it is not the way that children touch each other, it gives a strong message about appropriate behavior.

For the same reasons, children who are sexually provocative with adults also need a clear message back that their behavior is not okay. Sometimes kids behave in a sexual way inappropriate to their age because they want to know if all adults will take advantage of them.

Children who have been abused may also masturbate, looking for your response and because they like the feeling. Set your own family boundaries without making the child feel guilty.

I know sometimes your feelings become more than you think you can handle.

I know it can be real scary when you feel fine and then terrible. The terrible feelings will pass.

We can draw the things that scare you/that make you feel good.

Here is some clay you can pound while you are feeling mad.

I know a grownup did this to you, and you are mad about it, but I can't let you show your anger by taking it out on other kids.

You shouldn't steal another person's privacy, any more than you should steal candy from a store.

It isn't okay to do to someone else what happened to you.

Not all adults are sexual with kids, like Xxxxx. I'm not going to do that to you. This is a safe place.

It isn't okay at our house to flirt with adult men. They will pay attention to you without that. French kissing an adult is not okay.

It isn't okay to masturbate in the living room, but it is okay in your bedroom.

You can take a hot bath, play dress up, go shoot some baskets, or curl up in your bed instead.

CONTROL

Kids who have been abused are struggling to regain control over their environment. That is the developmental job of a child. Anything you can do to help your child feel more in control will help her/him feel better. This is usually a much bigger problem for children than the sexual concerns parents sometimes focus on.

Gaining control, for a child, means being able to listen to her/himself, feeling strong rather than helpless, being able to make some choices and trust feelings.

IS MY CHILD EVER GOING TO BE OKAY?

Recovering from sexual abuse is not smooth and level, but more like a roller coaster. Sometimes the angry outbursts, nightmares, or other behaviors can be triggered by seeing the abuser again, or having to go to court, going to counseling, seeing something on TV, or other reminders of the abuse.

A child who seems "worse" can actually be doing better. For instance, it might be that the child is not holding so much inside, being so guarded that she/he is denying all feelings. She/he is finding a way to express them to you. A child who seems to be over it, who then falls back into some of these behaviors, is a child who is trying to deal with and understand what happened. That's not bad; it needs to occur.

Your child will probably not be the same as before the abuse, but will certainly be able to get on with life. No one really stays the same anyway. Growing up implies continual change. You can look forward to your child stabilizing, especially if she/he is receiving treatment from a professional versed in child sexual abuse. Stabilized means your child has returned to kid activities, and has resolved as much as she/he can at this age about the abuse.

All this takes time. Each child needs to be able to take her/his own time. The child will be processing the abuse at each new developmental stage.

My Body Belongs to Me Activity

Let's get a large piece of butcher paper and tape it to the wall. Then you stand against the wall and I will trace all around your body. This might tickle a little. We can stop if you want. Think of the picture as divided into two sides; on one half you will be saying what you like, on the other half what you don't like. Start at the top of the drawing and fill in pictures answering the following questions about the body. You will have your own ideas, too, so we don't have to answer every question here.

What I like to be thinking is:	What I don't like to be thinking:
With my eyes I like to see:	With my eyes I don't like to see:
With my ears I like to hear:	With my ears I don't like to hear:
With my nose I like to smell:	With my nose I don't like to smell:
With my mouth I like to taste:	With my mouth I don't like to taste:
What makes my heart happy:	What makes my heart sad:
What makes my stomach smile:	What makes my stomach feel icky:
With my hands I like to touch:	With my hands I don't like to touch:
What makes my knees buckle:	What makes my knees stay straight:
What makes my feet want to run:	What makes my feet strong like a tree:

If the picture could say anything to anybody, what would it say? To whom would it say it? Write your answer on the picture.

Fill in hair, nose, eyes, mouth, clothes, etc. Give this picture some life.

Children's Reactions and Everyday Life
61

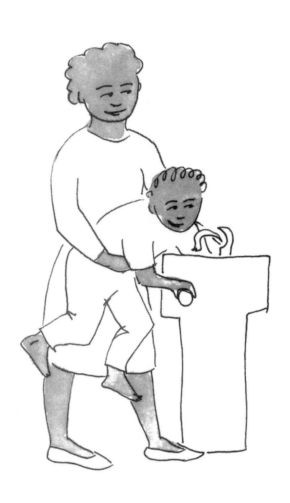

Chapter 5

Grieving . . . *"I'm crying but I can still take care of you"*

"At first I just went around in a fog. I did what I had to do, staying 'on hold,' locked in 'auto pilot.' I guess I was in shock those first weeks.

"I can't sleep. I don't cry. It's hard to fix a meal for myself. I feel sometimes as if I might explode. But I don't want my daughter to see me break down. I'm being strong for her sake."

"I never felt as though I could kill someone before. I think all the time about what I would do to this guy if I had him alone in a room. I'm having trouble at work. I sit down to do my work and suddenly it's two hours later and I don't know where the time went."

All I could do for a long time was to blame myself. I felt like a failure as a parent."

"At times I think the children are doing better than I am. Not many days go by that I don't think about it."

After a while, when my child began to sleep through the night without nightmares and the worst of the interviews were over, I had some time to think about what had happened. One night I started to cry. I was afraid I might never stop crying once I began. But after a couple hours I was all cried out. I expect I'll cry again."

AT FIRST

Catastrophes make us go numb. In that numb or shocked stage, we do what we have to do to get through it, and not much else.

It's likely to be sapping enormous energy from you as you try to "keep it all together." Add that to trouble sleeping, and its a wonder that you've been functioning at all. Many times the feeling is that if you do begin to show your feelings, you will "lose it," fall apart, not be able to stop crying or not be there for your child. Your anger may have fueled you up to this point. Now other reactions may be surfacing.

For parents, the sexual abuse of their child is a terrible loss. Most have lost a sense of the world as a safe place, or their home as a place of security, or their faith in the criminal justice system. You are feeling your losses, and you are going to be grieving for a while.

Grieving parents have expressed feelings of:

- enormous and overwhelming guilt
- anger, rage, revenge, sadness
- shame, disgust, embarrassment
- failure as parents
- sorrow at their child's loss of "innocence"
- knot, pain, ache in their stomach, or other physical reactions
- not being able to foresee a time when they may feel normal again
- loss of confidence in their ability to parent

I'm here with you.

I'll take care of you. I will keep you safe.

I can comfort you when you are sad. I can help you let you anger out.

Ask me when you want:
   a hug
   to be held
   to sit together.

I won't tell you what you <u>should</u> be feeling. I won't tell you to forget it.

I know this takes time. We can be patient together.

Sometimes you have to hurt for a while before you begin to feel better.

FOR YOURSELF

Find support. Parents of sexually abused children, in particular, are asked to put their own feelings aside and concentrate on being a support to the child. It isn't easy to do if you have no support yourself. Surround yourself with friends and family who are not critical; join a support group or see a counselor. If the sexual abuse was incest, it is even more important that you get support for yourself, since many people will be especially critical of you: "You must have known." "You weren't satisfying your husband sexually." "There must be something wrong with you for not knowing, or denying what was right in front of you."

Take the time to be alone. Find the time to cry. One mother said that she found the time by crying every time she did dishes. One father says that he pounds the racquetball harder and harder, pretending it is the abuser. It helps to schedule a time to grieve; clear a space for it. It is probably easier in the long run if you do your grieving from the beginning, instead of holding it all in.

Don't lose, in the crisis, your usual stress outlets, such as exercise, reading a mystery novel, taking a hot bath, gardening, watching TV. Yanking out weeds, digging, or chopping wood can be good outlets for grief and anger

Parents whose children have been abused often feel as though they are failures, that what happened was their fault. Most parents notice some of the effects of sexual abuse before the child discloses the abuse. Remember that no one should have to expect that sexual abuse has happened to their child. Finding out about the abuse may help you to understand health problems your child was having that seemed to be a mystery. You may be able to set the time of the onset of the abuse. It may help you to understand what signs you could have seen and why you didn't know. Many good parents have seen red spots on their child's neck and called them fleabites, and then been surprised and embarrassed when the child was sent home from school with a note saying she has chicken pox. Parents cannot be expected to know all and see all, and to never make mistakes.

I can handle it, whatever you are feeling. It won't upset me if you say something you think I don't want to hear. You don't need to take care of me that way.

What do you think will happen if you tell me what you are thinking? Do you think I will be angry? Do you think I will fall apart? What do you think falling apart means? That I would yell and yell until my throat was sore? That I would stop taking care of you? Even if I did fall apart, I wouldn't fall apart forever. I can take care of you.

You may feel bad or sad now. That's okay. You won't always feel this sad. I feel sad that it happened too, but I can still take care of you, and hear about your feelings. I'm sad that this happened to you. Sometimes that's how life is, being sad.

You do not need to take care of me. I'm an adult. I can take care of me. I'm your parent. I can take care of you.

Where do you feel sad? My feelings feel stuck in my throat. We could make a plan. We could decide to let out one sad (scary, stuck, bad) thing every day.

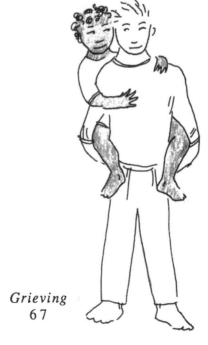

Grieving
6 7

WHY DID IT HAPPEN? WHY MY CHILD?

It didn't happen because of you or because of your child. It happened because the offender decided to do it. A lot of time can be spent trying to figure out what you might have done if only. . . . But blaming yourself for not suspecting the abuser or blaming your child for not telling or not resisting is counterproductive. Place the blame where it belongs, with the abuser. Child sexual abuse brings with it a terrible feeling of helplessness. Sometimes we imagine there were things we could have done just to avoid feeling helpless.

If you are in a two-parent home, stress of this kind causes troubles in relationships. Sometimes there are clashes of coping styles between one parent and another. One mother, for instance, felt it was sinful for her husband to feel that he would like to kill the molester, a teenage boy baby-sitter. She felt that her husband's expressed aggression was frightening. He thought she was being too forgiving of the offender. Sometimes differences in coping methods like these can cause a split between the couple. Each partner needs to recognize that the other may have an entirely different way of dealing with the sexual abuse of the child. It doesn't mean one response is better than another. They are just different.

HOW CAN MY CHILD GRIEVE THE LOSS OF SOMEONE WHO DID SOMETHING SO AWFUL?

Although many children feel only relief when the abuser is no longer part of daily life, it can be a source of pain if the offender was a close relative or friend. It is hard for children to understand that you can love someone yet not be able to live with him, or still have to hold him responsible for the sexual abuse. It helps children to understand if you separate the person from his actions. You didn't like what he did, although you like him.

This issue comes up again if the child is permitted to visit an abusing parent who has gone through treatment. Kids don't know whether they love or hate him. They need help in resolving these feelings or help in knowing that it is okay to wait and see how they feel about him.

I know you miss Xxxxx.

I miss him, too.

I feel badly about missing him when what he did was so bad.

But I don't miss the bad stuff. I miss the good stuff, like when he took us all for rides on the motor scooter.

It's okay to like someone, and be angry at them.

You can still love someone, even though they have a serious problem. Sometimes that problem means you can't live with them, though.

I know it took me a long time to understand this.

REMEMBERING YOUR OWN ABUSE

Sometimes parents remember being abused themselves when the sexual abuse of their child is disclosed. Abuse in childhood leaves you with a special vulnerability. Your feelings and responses to your own child's abuse may be more intense. Don't let your memories of abuse trigger you into the powerlessness of your own childhood victimization. Instead, take care of that hurting child within you.

Find some help: If you haven't already, seek out counselors who specialize in treatment of adults who were molested as children. Make sure your counselor has had training in this area.

1. Find a trusted person you can tell about what happened to you.

2. Read a book written for adults who were molested as children.

3. Keep notes as your own memories surface. You do not need to be rushed by others into confronting your abuser until you have done more healing: before you are ready, before you have outside help, before you are prepared for the denial.

4. If it was the same person who abused your child and you, then both you and your child should get outside help.

5. Don't get locked into multigenerational guilt—that because you were abused, your kids were more at risk, that since you were abused yourself you should have known the signs better. Remember that it takes people willing to take advantage for abuse to happen.

6. Decide whether or not you want to talk with your child about your abuse. Know that your child's experience is almost certainly different from your own. Look at all the ways her/his childhood is not like yours. Look at the ways your response to the abuse has been different.

7. Add the grieving of your own losses to the grieving of your child's. Grieve the loss of the relationship (or the ideal of the relationship) whether it was husband, father, grandfather, brother, friend, or neighbor.

8. Accept that the recovery process will go on for a long time. Bits and pieces of the past will come up at different times in your life.

I'm sorry it happened to you.

Even though I had a similar experience myself, I know it's not the same for you as it was for me.

I have my own feelings, so do you. They don't have to be the same. They are all important.

You and I can get through this together.

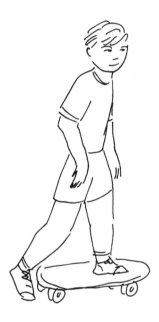

CHILDREN GRIEVE TOO

You will need to give your child permission to talk about the pain. Children want so much to protect you, or not upset you, that they sometimes keep their true feelings inside. They will especially keep feelings suppressed if it seems you can't handle it. They feel they need to take care of you.

Sometimes boys need more encouragement to talk about and express their feelings than girls do. Boys are raised with less permission to feel bad, feel used, or feel ashamed than we give girls. Boys are often raised to be tough and to be able to handle themselves, and not cry or lose control. A boy may feel especially burdened with the need to take care of his mother if incest happened and the father or father figure is now out of the home. Boys sometimes try to make up your loss for you, thinking every home needs a man to be safe. Don't let your child take on this role.

Children are sometimes afraid to talk about the sexual abuse to their parents, afraid they will make their parent cry. A counselor would ask the child "What would happen if what you told made your mom cry? Will she fall apart?" They need your encouragement to let the feelings out.

Children's feelings can stay "stuck" inside them. One little girl said she could feel them sitting in her stomach. She said she knew they could move up and out her mouth, so she held her mouth tightly shut. She had no one who made it safe and secure for her to talk. Your child needs to know that you can handle whatever she has to say, because if you can't, how can she?

It is important that you help your child grieve. Children grieve as actively as adults do, whether you see it or not. Withdrawal, anxiety, aggressiveness, anger, despair, and sadness are all signs of a child's grief.

I see you are looking out the window again. Sometimes I do that too.

You seem depressed today. Are you?

I feel anxious or worried about going to work now, just as you feel anxious about going to school. That's normal.

You're really mad at me right now. You seem to be having lots of strong feelings.

I can take the time to:
> listen to you
> be with you
> cuddle and hold you.

Let's talk about crying. What are some reasons people cry?
Because they're sad, hurt, scared, frustrated, happy, tired, moved.

You are not a sissy if you cry. You won't always feel this bad.
Everyone has those feelings sometimes. Sometimes that's how life is, being sad.

You may think I never cry. But I do, even if you don't see me. It's okay for mommies (or daddies) and for little girls (or boys) to cry.

I cry because this hurts me too. But I can take care of you. Because I'm crying too doesn't mean I'm falling apart. I'm crying but can still take care of you. I'm not crying because of anything you did.

If you hear me crying, it's all right. It makes me feel better to cry. You can cry too.

SIGHING

Sighing is a sign of grief. Other signs are tense muscles, sleeplessness, getting sick frequently, and behaving differently.

Set aside a time to grieve together. For example, go to a movie with some sad scenes and cry together. It's not necessary to tell the child that this is a time to grieve. You might just say nothing and enjoy the relief from a good cry, or you might say to your child, "It feels better just to cry sometimes."

AFTER SOME TIME

After the immediate crisis has passed, and you have settled into a routine, and you think that now is the time for you to start to feel better, it's not unusual to get depressed.

You may be feeling tired, lethargic, having trouble concentrating, trouble sleeping, or getting out of bed in the morning. You may not feel like eating or you may be eating compulsively; you may have lost your sex drive. These are normal feelings when you are grieving. These are signs that say loud and clear that you have suffered a loss.

You don't feel better, and you think you should. The hurt isn't going away. The legal system, the other professionals, didn't relieve the pain. This is a normal reaction to stress. What you are feeling only makes sense. You've put your needs on "hold" for so long. Now that things have calmed down a bit, it is only natural for your own needs to surface, and for you to have feelings of grief and loss at having your world shattered.

If you have held it all in until legal proceedings are over and the pressures are less, you are likely to experience more exaggerated feelings than if you had experienced them every day. Opening the floodgates may cause you to feel you're going to drown. But the feelings are the same. You have the right to grieve for your child and yourself and the past and the losses. It will take more time to grieve your losses if the abuser was close to you.

I can't take your pain away, but I can help.

We can name feelings: happy, sad, angry, afraid. Let's write them on cards and stick them on the fridge when you are feeling that way.

It's okay to have those feelings.

When you slam the door, I know you must be feeling angry.

Maybe you don't want to cry in front of anyone. Sometimes it helps to set aside a time to cry, like when you are in the bathroom.

I have some special cardboard boxes/blocks here. I thought you might want to stack them all up, and then knock them all down. I used to do that when I was a boy. It helped me when I was mad.

Here is a hammer and some nails set in a board. Pounding on them can help you get that anger out.

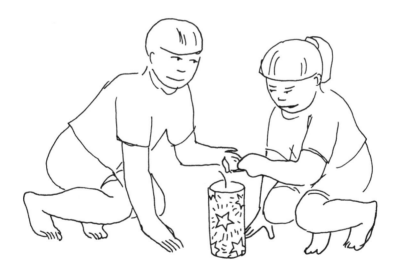

Grieving

FOR YOURSELF

Short-term counseling for yourself and/or your spouse may be in order. There is no point in suffering alone when talking with a counselor could help.

Take good care of yourself. (Take a hot bath to relax, for example.) You are not taking care of yourself if you are smoking or drinking too much, not exercising, taking tranquilizers, not eating, or eating too much junk food.

Try to reword some of the depressing and negative messages that are going around in your mind. For example, change "I'll never trust again" to "I am going to change the way I trust people, and find new ways." Change "I'm a bad parent" to "No parent is perfect, or knows everything, or sees everything, or is all powerful." Change "My child will never be the same" to "Change is a part of living. Children are sturdy and resilient." Change "It will always be like this" to "The only way from here is up" or "There are lots of little things we do each day that are getting us back to normal."

Know that it will get better with time. You've suffered a loss. This loss triggers grieving you didn't do when you suffered other losses in your life. (One mother said, "Why do I hate my ex-husband so much now—the divorce was ten years ago." She was very confused that her main reaction to the current problem was that she hated her ex-husband.)

You may begin to feel better one week only to find yourself falling apart thinking about the abuse again the next day. You may be replaying the events of the sexual abuse over and over in your head, driving away anyone who is close to you, feeling as if you are a new person and wanting the old one back. Pain and grief come in waves. You can think to yourself: it will pass—I know I can wait until the wave passes.

Your child is going through the same process. If your child is sad and angry for a long time (over a year if the loss was major) or if your child doesn't express any feelings, it is important to get her/him extra help.

A Read-Together Story:

HEIDI THE DOG

David had a dog named Heidi. Heidi could walk on her hind feet and bark, but David loved her especially because she was always there when he came home from school, she always wanted to play, and she always wanted to be cuddled. David and Heidi were special friends, even though some days David would rather do something else besides taking Heidi for her walk and couldn't stand the thought of having to feed her, or getting yelled at if he forgot.

One day, on a walk, David took Heidi to the store to buy some milk for his mother. He tied her leash on a post outside the door, and told her to stay. She was used to that, as David often walked to the store for his mother.

But when he came out of the store, Heidi was gone! He kept thinking that if he blinked his eyes, she would be back at the post, where he left her. David asked everyone outside the store if they had seen Heidi. People told him that Heidi had bitten someone, and the dogcatcher had come and taken Heidi. David went home without Heidi, because he knew his mother would be worried. His mom called the dogcatcher, but they said they didn't have her.

David felt different without Heidi. He wasn't as happy. He missed the fun things they used to do together, although he didn't miss having to feed and walk her everyday. It was hard not knowing where Heidi was, and what had happened to her. He wondered if Heidi missed him as much as he missed her. David felt as though it was his fault that she was lost—if only he hadn't gone to the store that day, or if only he hadn't had bad feelings about feeding her everyday, it wouldn't have happened.

It was hard and sad for David to lose such a good friend. David cried a lot, when he needed to. It hurts to lose a friend. But it helps to talk about it with someone. What would you say to David if he could talk to you?

Chapter 6

Rebuilding Self-Esteem . . . *"It wasn't your fault"*

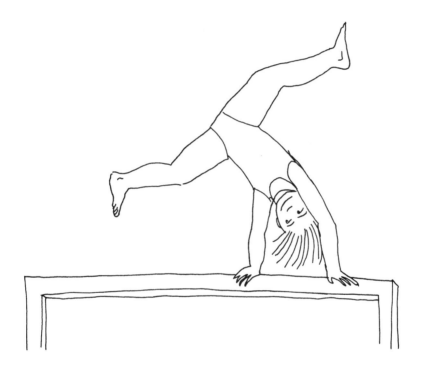

SOMETIMES BAD THINGS HAPPEN TO GOOD PEOPLE

Abused children don't feel as good about themselves as children who have not been victimized. Children with lower self-esteem don't do as well in school, are hesitant about new activities, making friends, and don't expect to be treated well. Parents can rebuild self-esteem by helping children understand that

they are not "bad" because they were abused,

they are not at fault,

they do not need to feel ashamed, different, or isolated.

Children may come to the conclusion they are bad because they believe:

Bad things happen to bad people

Sex is bad

Bad things happen to me when I am bad

I feel bad, so I must be bad.

You are working against children's beliefs as you help them understand that the abuse did not happen because they were "bad." To help children understand rules, adults often make statements linking a child's misbehavior to a later painful outcome: "I told you if you went barefoot, you would cut your foot."

When children are sexually abused, they usually expect to be blamed. They may even think adults knew what was happening, and let it continue because they were being punished.

Do you believe that bad things only happen to bad people?"

Let's write NOT TRUE right across the top of that.

Sometimes bad things happen to good children. It isn't fair, but it happens.

Children are not responsible for controlling other people, especially adults.

If children knew everything adults knew, they wouldn't be children.

Adults are responsible for controlling their own behavior. It would be wrong for an adult to steal something, even if a kid asked him to. The adult should know better. If an adult tricks a child, the adult is the one at fault.

You did the best you could, with what you knew.

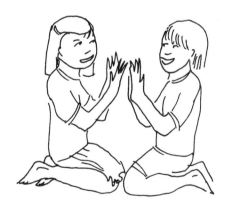

Rebuilding Self-Esteem

FEELINGS

You can sit down with your child and talk about her/his feelings, without arguing or trying to change her/his mind. Parents have a very hard time when children feel bad and want to make them feel better. Children can learn from this pressure to feel good that bad feelings aren't allowed, or that they are bad because they have bad feelings. You can suggest some other ways your child could act out feelings.

If your child expresses confusion about feelings, or positive feelings about the offender, you can listen and reassure her/him those are normal feelings.

Probably the most frightening emotion is intense anger, wishing someone dead or worse. Your child may or may not have trouble admitting anger and the thoughts that go with it. You can help by stating your own anger and acknowledging that sometimes it is frightening, but that you can handle yours and hers/his.

Crummy feelings don't make you crummy.

What are some of the reasons you might feel crummy?
    You think no one believed you?
    You wish you had been able to do something?
    You think we are disappointed in you?
    You hurt inside?
    Someone you love and trusted hurt you?

You are not bad because you are mad. I might not let you hurt another child, but you are not bad because you sometimes feel like hurting someone.

There are other ways to express that angry feeling:
    Draw a picture of that person and tear it up, or put it on a dart board.
    Write a note to him you never send about being mad.
    Go outside and get some exercise. Run real hard around the block.

It doesn't make you bad if you aren't mad either. You may have a whole bunch of feelings that don't agree. You might just be numb or mixed up.

Feelings aren't right or wrong. They just are.

CHILDREN MAY FEEL AT FAULT FOR WHAT THEY DIDN'T DO, OR WHAT THEY DID DO

Even adults are sometimes confused about why kids don't use self-protection rules. Both adults and children believe bad things only happen to other people, and ignore safety rules. Sometimes the rules don't work even when followed. Children should not be responsible for preventing sexual abuse. Adults should be. Whatever kids can do to protect themselves is great, but children do not have the understanding of the world necessary to ward off all danger from adults who want to take advantage of them.

You can help your children understand fault better by talking about what is their fault and what isn't. Examples of other things that adults are not supposed to do with kids may help them understand the difference in responsibility.

Your child may have said no and the offender didn't listen, or told her/him:

"You really like it or you wouldn't be here."

"If you haven't told already, who is going to believe you now?"

"You went along with it before, you can't get out of it now."

Fault

Some things are a child's fault. It's your fault if . . .

    you don't feed the dog when it is your chore

    you don't keep your room clean so you can't find your shoes

    you leave your jacket at the baseball field and don't find it until the next day after it rains

    you fail a test because you didn't study

It's <u>not</u> your fault if . . .

    you fail a test because something bad happened to you and you couldn't concentrate

    there's an earthquake

    your mother (or father, or stepmother, or grandmother, or baby sister) catches the flu

    you get tripped while you are running

    you're hungry before dinner time

    you do what an adult says, and then find out that he was tricking you

    you like special attention and like being held

SELF-BLAME

Children may blame themselves for something they did. Maybe they went back to the situation because they hoped he wouldn't do it again, they imagined it, or that they would be able to stop him this time. Maybe they believed the offender when he said he was sorry and he'd never do it again. Sometimes children feel stupid because someone tricked them or bribed them and they didn't know any better.

Children blame themselves for not telling, even though they thought they'd get into trouble for telling, or believed that they were protecting their parents by not telling. They may not understand why they didn't tell sooner, even though at the time they were terrorized by cruel and frightening threats or overwhelmed by an adult's authority.

SECRETS DAMAGE SELF ESTEEM

Children may identify themselves as victims, and pick up society's message that "victims are losers." They may feel unclean or used, and become ashamed and embarrassed about what happened to their bodies.

If they were keeping a secret, then every time they were praised they may have thought "if you knew, you wouldn't love me."

Even children who are too young to know what is wrong about abuse are sensitive to adults. They may sense from the atmosphere of secrecy that they should be ashamed.

Sometimes when you look back on something it looks really easy. Remember when you first learned to:

Tie your own shoes?

Ride your bike?

Button your own shirt?

You may not even remember how hard it was because it seems so easy now. Saying "no" sounds easy too. But I know most kids get through what happened to you by being numb. Looking back on how you were tricked or forced you could wonder why you didn't know what to do. But the first time you try to do something it can look so hard, it is too scary to try.

Being a victim is temporary.

You aren't a "loser" because the other person didn't play by the rules.

Is anyone a total "loser"? Someone whose team loses a soccer game could win next week. Everyone is a winner somehow.

Being tricked or bribed doesn't make you stupid. I bet there are other times in your life when you wished you had done something different, but it didn't turn out so badly.

Your body is not different. Nothing shows because you were sexually abused. No one will know who isn't told. Many other children have been abused. I know you can't tell who by looking.

I love you now, and I loved you when you were keeping the secret.

YOUR FAITH IN YOUR CHILD'S ABILITY TO HEAL AND RECOVER

Children regain confidence as they are able to do the same things other children their age do. After you have provided comfort, encourage your child to explore on her/his own, go bike riding, play baseball, have friends over, go to the library.

You can ask them to help with the household, and praise them for the completion of tasks. Ask for help fixing dinner, dressing a younger child, or deciding where to go for a picnic.

Deciding when to comfort and when to press for more mature behavior is sometimes difficult. A parenting class, a book, a counselor, friends, or grandparents can help you decide what is normal behavior for your child's age. For example, a seven year old who says that no one likes her could be suffering from shame over the abuse, but seven year olds typically go through a phase when they believe no one cares.

Children who become supercompetent need help understanding that they are valued just for being. These children need praise for a laugh, a smile, playing, or tears. You may want to say, "I'm glad you're here, and that you are who you are."

If children do adult chores, you can thank them and let them know you expect them to take some time just for themselves.

I really appreciate your help. Why don't you go do something you like to do, just for you.

Three Joys

Even though our life isn't exactly the way we want it to be right now, there are things that make us happy, or bring us joy if we notice them. Let's tell each other three joys each day.

Look for colors, shapes, or patterns you like. Notice smells, or sounds. See what textures feel good. Notice when other people do something you like. Remember when you do something during the day that makes you happy.

Then at dinner time or bedtime we can tell each other three fun, interesting, exciting, pretty, or new things about our day.

Here are some ideas:
> I enjoyed the sunset today.
> I learned a new way to do some of my work.
> I decided I like the color green again.

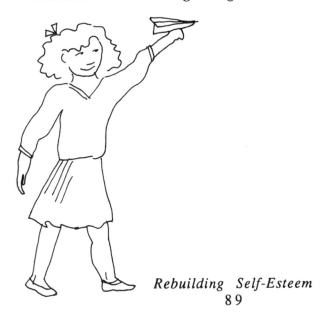

Rebuilding Self-Esteem

AFFIRMATIONS

Affirmations can be helpful for children to hear. Affirmations are different from praise. You can use affirmations even when your child's behavior is out of control. <u>Being</u> affirmations such as "I'm glad you are here" and "I like who you are" may be even more important in those circumstances than <u>doing</u> affirmations such as "I appreciate your help with the yard," "You worked hard on that book report," or "You really played well today." These statements may seem unnecessary because you think kids already know you love them and care about them no matter what happens to them. But you don't know what an offender has said or what the child may have picked up from magazines, newspapers, or TV about who is lovable.

Boys' and girls' self-esteem may be affected differently. Boys may feel the loss of power more, since power is viewed as an important male characteristic. Girls may fear the loss of lovability more. This is a time to develop a balanced picture. Usually girls get compliments for looks, being nice, taking care of others. Boys are praised for being smart, capable, adventuresome. Both boys and girls need compliments and praise.

Building your child's self-esteem means
   talking,
   touching,
   praising,
   expecting competency,
   trusting your child's ability to care for herself/himself,
   accepting feelings as valid but distinguishing between feelings and actions,
   being trustworthy and honest about what is happening,
   and modeling self-caring behavior.

AFFIRMATIONS are statements about strengths and positive wishes. These affirmations are from parents to kids:

I'm glad you are here.

I'm glad you are a boy/girl.

You can take as much time as you need to grow up.

It is okay to be scared and hurt.

It is okay to be powerful and responsible.

Your body is just fine.

It is powerful to know how to dress yourself, make friends, know what you like and don't like, ride a bike, climb a tree, take the bus, read a book, be able to find your way to school and back. Skills and abilities are power.

What Affirmations Would You Like to Make for Yourself?

State them in the positive: "I will be confident and sure of myself," rather than "I won't be scared."

You can affirm things you wish to become, because affirmations are a little bit of magic.

Chapter 7

Sexuality . . . *"You're still lovable"*

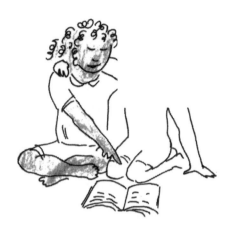

HELPING CHILDREN UNDERSTAND

Children, even preschoolers, need a gradual understanding or picture of what healthy sexuality is, to replace what the child learned through the abuse. Since it is hard to talk about sexuality and parents often lack basic information themselves, this may be the most difficult task of all. But children left on their own to puzzle through what happened are left vulnerable to further victimization. Many adults victimized as children suffer sexual difficulties. Providing children with accurate, understandable information about sexuality that does not add to their sense of shame or guilt may help avoid some of the later problems.

The goals are:

- Helping children develop the basic vocabulary to talk about sexuality

- Teaching children accurate information and socially acceptable sexual boundaries to replace the unhealthy ones taught by the offender

- Setting appropriate limits around sexual acting-out behavior

- Reducing the child's shame and confusion

After the immediate crisis is over, children need the language to talk about their bodies. If your child did not know the correct terms before the abuse, don't teach them until legal proceedings are complete. It could appear you had coached her/him.

I know it is going to be hard to start a conversation if you don't have the words. Here are body part words, let's match them.

	anus
	back
arm	breasts
	buttocks
	calf
	chest
genitals	clitoris
	ears
	eyes
	elbow
head	finger
	foot
	hand
	knee
trunk	mouth
	nose
	penis
	stomach
leg	testicles
	thigh
	vagina
	vulva

MY CHILD DOESN'T SEEM INTERESTED

Young children may seem to attach little or no sexual meaning to what happened to them. Other worries, fears, and betrayals, such as losing a friend or losing special treatment, may be more important to them. Sometimes this lack of sexual concern on a child's part can mislead a parent into thinking the child is not hurt or that sexuality doesn't need attention. But children who have been exposed to unhealthy sexual behavior need adult help to counter what was learned.

They may think they have a hole that shouldn't be there, or that their bodies are abnormal because of their response. A good sex education book is a useful tool for helping children gain the vocabulary they need to talk about what happened and ask questions about their own bodies. Without the tools and words, they can't ask about their confusion.

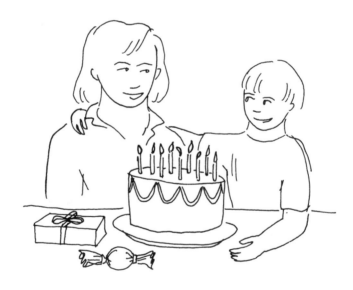

Sexuality
96

Your body is special. You deserve love.

Did you know that the feeling you get when you are excited about a soccer game is the same one you get when you're afraid of a dog? We call one excitement and the other fear, but to the body it is the same.

Have you ever laughed when you were embarrassed or scared? That's your body being confused, too, about what is going on.

You may be confused about what love is, what trust is, what sex is, what caring is. You have lots of time to learn more so you won't be confused.

You know how tickling feels good and is fun if you can stop the tickler when you want to. For example, you like to be tickled by Uncle John, but not by your cousin Sara.

Well sex is a little like that. It is okay, fun and feels good when it is what you want, the person cares for you and you for her/him, and you are both old enough to be responsible and make good decisions. Some people say this can happen only in marriage. In our family we believe_____.

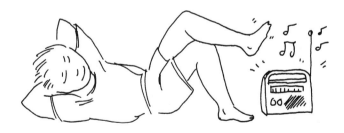

Sexuality

SETTING SOCIALLY ACCEPTABLE BOUNDARIES

Sexual abuse may create more difficulty when bribes, love, extra attention, or privileges were used. Children in these circumstances feel guilty about not resisting and getting something they wanted. They may say they weren't forced, no one made them do it, so if it is wrong, it is their fault.

Sometimes they appear to have learned that the way to get affection is by giving sex. For example, one little girl hopped up on men's laps and offered to give them kisses.

This child needs to be taken aside and given reasonable limits, and helped to find other acceptable ways to get attention.

School-age girls may experiment with clothes to test attractiveness, to test seductiveness, to find a way to be sexy now that the abuse has ended. You needn't let your eight-year old child dress as if she is sixteen, but do let her dress the way other eight year olds are dressing. You needn't allow seductive behavior. You can simply say it isn't okay behavior with adults. (Say it privately.) Some sexual abuse victims seem to test the adults around them to "prove" that adults are all like that, or because they had some measure of power within an abuse situation.

Children may need reassurance that wanting to cuddle and touch is normal and healthy, and that they deserve nurturing, affectionate touching.

You don't have to share your body. You are lovable the way you are.

Children aren't old enough to have to decide if what the adult is asking is okay. Adults are supposed to know. An adult who has sexual contact with a child is being unfair, breaking the rules no matter what he gives the child. The child isn't wrong for liking what she/he was given.

Children are supposed to be protected from having to guess, because it is too hard for children to say no to adults, especially if they offer something you really want.

It isn't okay at our house to flirt with adult men. They will pay attention to you without that. French kissing with an adult is not okay.

Someone promised you, even if it wasn't in words, something too big to turn down, but he asked you for something you shouldn't have had to give. It is too high a price to pay.

Now I want to help you find other ways to get what you want other than trading kisses. You deserve love and attention without trading anything. Special treats and privileges are earned. Do you have some ideas how you can do that? You can ask for what you want. You can do a chore, or earn some money for a special favor. What are some other ideas?

We all like and need hugs and pats from people who love and care about us. You can ask for a hug and get one, "no strings attached."

SETTING LIMITS

Sexual abuse increases the confusion parents experience around sexual issues. Because you want to allow children healthy sexuality and to protect your child from shame, you may not be certain what behavior should be stopped. Children are dependent on adults to provide information about behavior in general and especially sexual behavior.

You may need to say to your child, "I know that feels good to you, but you cannot (lie on top of your sister and rub on her, be sexual with the dog, kiss daddy that way, masturbate in the living room). You may want to help your child find other ways to gain comfort and pleasure acceptable to you.

Sexual exploration between siblings, such as playing doctor, is normal. If you encounter your children in such exploration, suggest some rules:

No one else can join in.

If someone says no you must stop.

No objects, not even a tongue depressor, are to be used in the play.

Children are to be in a safe place.

They must be close to the same age.

If either child appears to be sexually aggressive or is using an object, that is not normal exploration and signals a need for help. Children sometimes act out on other children what happened to them. Find a specialist in treating victims of child sexual abuse who understands how to work with these acting-out behaviors.

We've been talking about confusion. Let's talk about what our house rules are.

If you feel bad, talk to me.

It is okay to find a way to have good feelings, but we have rules about how you can do it.

It isn't okay to masturbate in the living room, but it is okay in your bedroom.

You can take a hot bath, play dress up, go shoot some baskets, curl up on your bed.

What ideas can you think of?

It can be confusing to separate sexual feelings from affectionate feelings. You deserve affectionate touching and loving without sexual touching.

Can you draw a picture of the confusion we are all feeling? What color is it? What animal is it?

Maybe what you really want is some cuddling and affection. You can ask for that too. You can sit down next to me and we can cuddle. Or ask for a neck massage. I can say no or yes too, just as you can.

REDUCING CHILDREN'S SHAME AND CONFUSION.

Most children are very confused about sex.

One girl said, "My mother always told me that sex with love was beautiful. I didn't love him, so what I did was dirty and awful."

This child, like many others, needs help understanding that what she did wasn't her responsibility. The adult was wrong.

Because sex is often associated with being "bad," you will need to continue to talk with your child to help her/him understand that she/he is not bad because of the abuse.

Sexual abuse is harmful to a child's developing sexuality because of the associations children learn. They may learn that the only way people show love or caring is through sex. They may learn that sex is equal to fear. They may grow up damaged in learning how to trust.

Sexual abuse is harmful because it stimulates children in a powerful way for which they have no outlet after abuse ends. Some kids numb their bodies and feelings just to survive the abuse. Others numb their bodies later. Some repeatedly seek risky sexual experiences, preferring the excitement that comes from taking a risk to other feelings.

Sometimes the stimulation in abuse situations feels good, while the rest of the situation feels bad. Bodies may respond even when the stimulation is unwanted. This can be very confusing to children.

An offender increases a child's confusion when he responds to a child's protest with, "It feels good doesn't it." Or "It's normal for kids to do this and like it." Then when the abuse is disclosed, the child learns it wasn't normal, and may decide she/he must be weird because it felt good.

He tricked you. He knew better. He may have told you lies.

Sometimes adults who do this tell kids funny or strange things that are hard to understand. These are "lines." Lines can confuse us about what we really think. Everyone gets fooled sometimes by a line. You've heard your aunt say, "What a line . . . ." Well, that's what she means. Sometimes you can see them for what they are, but other times it is really hard.

Maybe he said something like:

> *"I just want to teach you about sex."*
>
> *"It feels good doesn't it."*
>
> *"You really do want it."*
>
> *"What's the matter, don't you trust me?"*
>
> *"This is how people show each other they love them."*
>
> *"You'll do this some day anyway."*
>
> *"Let's play we are married."*

These are lines. Some are lies, some are just confusing and tricky.

Did Xxxxx say anything confusing that you want to ask me about?

PROVIDE INFORMATION

Children need reassurances that the way their bodies responded was normal. Without adult help, they have no way to make sense of the sexual experiences. They can't talk about it with their friends, and if adults don't bring it up, they believe it can't be talked about. It remains secret and shameful and the child's recovery is partially blocked. If the abuse was by an offender of the same sex the child may be concerned about being homosexual. Sexual abuse means nothing about sexual preference. The adult picked the situation, not the child. Providing your child with age-appropriate sex education is the best way to help develop healthy sexuality.

Examples explaining the difference between sexual abuse and wanted sex are best put in terms of their experiences.

Your child may need help separating simple touch and sex. Your child should have the right to stop touching when it becomes uncomfortable. But parents need to keep touching their children. Children need hugs, cuddles, and physical contact. They need to know that some touch comes without any sexual strings attached. If the child looks uncomfortable, try saying something like "This is just a hug" before letting go.

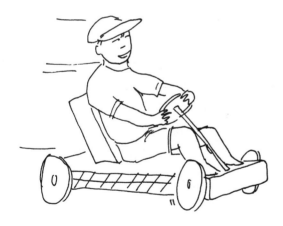

Sexuality

A Story

Once a little boy really wanted to go fishing with his dad. But
when his dad woke him up at five in the morning he was mad.
He wanted to sleep. He hadn't known they were going to get up so
early, and it was cold. As he sat in the boat and the sun started to
warm him, he felt better but he wondered why they couldn't have
waited to come. He couldn't ask his dad though, because he feared
his dad would tease him about being a baby. He didn't know
whether to have fun or be mad. He felt tricked and trapped in the
boat, but he liked the sunshine and being with his dad.

When Thoughts and Feelings Conflict

Your body can be telling you one thing (this feels good), while your
mind tells you something else (this isn't right) and your feelings tell
you something else again (this is icky, embarrassing, frightening).

Your mind can be asking: "Is this right?"

Your feelings may be: sad, or happy, or angry

At the same time your body may be feeling: hot, or cold, or pain, or
pleasure.

When sex works right (when you are older)- your mind, body and
feelings are close together.. You know the rules and the consequences,
and you take care of yourself and are careful of the other person. Your
body feels good, your feelings are pleasant.

You can tell me not to hug you right now.

I'm not going to ask for anything else from you. There are no strings
attached to this hug.

Chapter 8

Self-Protection . . . *"Never again"*

"I'm going to be very cautious for quite a while. Like most people, I never really thought it could happen to my kids."

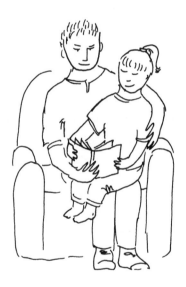

LEARNING TO FEEL SAFE

Helping your child to feel safer, to know when to trust, to feel stronger, and feel better about herself, to feel in control of her body, to know how to get positive attention, is all part of her recovery process. It also helps the child protect her/himself against further abuse.

Sexual abuse can happen to any child, and about 50% of abused kids are abused again. Statistically, it appears that some sexual abuse victims continue to be victimized throughout their lives, in different ways. It isn't known why—perhaps because of feelings that they don't deserve any better or because the studies deal with adults who never got any help as children.

As long as child sexual abuse is a reality, it makes sense to try to help children protect themselves. Actually, all of this book concerns helping children prevent sexual abuse in the future, since the more they understand about sexual abuse, and the better they feel about themselves, the less likely they are to be confused or frightened, or to keep the secret. This chapter concerns specific actions you can take to better your child's self-protection abilities.

There are, however, no guarantees. Teaching kids to recognize and respond to sexual abuse provides some chance of reducing their vulnerability. If we are to prevent sexual abuse, we must create a society without sexual offenders.

While you teach your children self-protection, repeat to them that it is not their fault if they can't or didn't do what you suggest. It shouldn't be up to children in the first place to get adults to do what's right. It is not fair to hold children totally responsible for protecting themselves. We sometimes forget they are only children and that stopping a determined adult is hard.

Affirmations

It's okay to try things, start things, be curious, be alert. You can get support and protection at the same time.

You can both think and feel. You can use both to decide things.

You can be sure about what you need.

I'm glad you are growing up.

You can be powerful and still have needs.

You can be taken care of even when you aren't frightened, sick, sad, or mad.

You can express your feelings straight.

CHILD SEXUAL ABUSE PREVENTION EDUCATION

<u>Cautions for using prevention books and videos with a child who has been abused</u>: If you are reading a prevention book with your child, take care that its messages are ones that will not add to your child's sense of failure for having not "prevented" abuse in the past. Most sexual abuse prevention education programs have been developed for children who have not been abused, and may not be sensitive to children who have already been abused.

ASK YOURSELF

- Does the book (video, comic) imply that all abuse is preventable? It isn't, and it isn't a child's responsibility either.

- Does the book make it clear whose fault the abuse is? Some say nothing about that.

- Does it use judgmental language? (For example, you *should* say no, you *must* tell, it's *good* to do this. This tends to add to the child's burden of guilt. Kids think "I should have said no," "I failed because I didn't, or because the abuser didn't listen," I'm bad because I didn't tell," "I'm stupid because I didn't run away".)

- Does it deny them the support or help of adults? It does not reassure kids to think they will have to face dangerous or threatening situations alone; it's not fair to expect that of them.

- Does it overemphasize the danger of strangers? Prevention teaching should aim at reducing fears, not increasing them. Stranger danger messages are likely to do the opposite. Also, it was probably not a stranger who abused your child.

It is important that any self-protection training you do with your child does not add to your child's burden of guilt.

I know you did what the book said to do and he abused you anyway.

It's not up to children to get adults to do what is right.

It's not your fault that he didn't listen.

It's not your fault if you weren't able to say anything or get away.

Adults should know better than to trick kids.

The prevention book was my way of talking to you about sexual abuse. I'm glad it helped you to tell me.

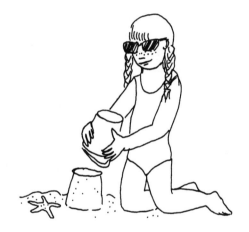

SELF-PROTECTION

Children who have been abused need special help to feel safe again, to stand up for themselves, to feel good about themselves and their bodies, to expect good treatment from others, to know what persons to trust, and to ask for help with problems. These are the basic foundations of self-protection.

TRUST

Abuse extended over a long time teaches children the wrong things about trust: "Those I trust aren't trustworthy," or "I don't have the ability to know who to trust; there must be something wrong with me." "I can't trust my feelings."

Trust is a difficult issue, even for adults. Some mothers of children who have been sexually abused can also recall many instances of personal betrayals, to the point where they are wondering if they will ever find a trustworthy man. People are trustworthy to varying degrees and in different ways, so there are no perfect answers.

As tempting as it is to offer <u>stranger danger</u> information insisting that children trust no one outside the family, that does not prepare children (especially teenagers) to go out on their own. Or, since most child sexual abuse is by someone known, parents feel they must decide to trust no person ever again. It is an impossible stance to never trust anyone again, to always be in control of what happens to your child. It can't be done.

Kids needs tools and life skills, not generalizations.

It is much more useful to help children learn to trust themselves and their feelings about people and situations and to understand that we learn to trust people who treat us with respect.

Most adults are not like Xxxxx. Most will help you if they know you are in danger. Most adults and teenagers are trustworthy.

Feelings

You can't tell about people by the way they look. So how do you know? You can trust your feelings. If someone is making you uncomfortable, you are right. Listen to these feelings. How do you decide who to trust? Is it a person you like? People who talk to you? I think the most important thing you can do is pay attention to your feelings about a person.

Behavior

Let's talk about who you can trust and why: He listens. He's never asked me to keep a secret. He also stops when I say to stop (tickling, wrestling, teasing). People are trustworthy when their talk and their actions match up. People who can be trusted are willing to try to understand, instead of making fun of your concerns. They treat you well.

Maybe we could start talking about the people you know you can't trust:
- People who ask you to keep secrets, not just private stuff like surprises, but secrets
- People who promise something for nothing
- People who try to come into the house when there isn't another adult home
- Kids who drink and drive
- Adults who drink and drive
- Adults who tell you something is all right when you've been taught it is wrong
- People who ask to take your picture without any clothes on
- People who offer you drugs
- People who try to blackmail you or trick you by saying they will tell your parents if you don't do something
- People who give you special favors and try to get you alone

Self-Protection

BODY RIGHTS

Children learn to ignore their own feelings in uncomfortable situations, instead of recognizing them as warnings. You can help children by telling them "If you think it feels funny or strange, you are right" and that it's okay to act on that feeling of discomfort. You can help children to know that they have a right to make some decisions about their bodies.

It is easiest for children to learn this by the way they live this. Respecting their boundaries at home gives them a strong sense of what those boundaries are, and that other people shouldn't cross them without permission. This means doing things such as knocking before going into a child's room, understanding when kisses to grandma are too uncomfortable and helping the child find a polite alternative, and respecting a child's personal "space." All family members deserve this respect, but it is of particular help to sexually abused children because most have had their personal boundaries invaded repeatedly.

Your body belongs to you. You can decide who touches it.

You can make decisions about your body.

If someone wants to pat your bottom, you can tell them not to.

Your feelings will tell you when things don't seem quite right. Listen to your feelings.

You deserve privacy when you need it.

I'll stop tickling you when you ask me to.

I'll tell you when I don't like certain touches, and you can too.

You are safe with me. I'm not going to abuse you.

I'd just like to give you a hug, no strings attached.

PRIVACY

Children need a way to reclaim their bodies for themselves. Since bath time, bedtime, and getting dressed may have been when abuse took place, building safe rituals around them may help children reclaim their space. Those abused at home lose the very security of their own beds. Nowhere is safe for them.

Bath time can be a good time, with younger children who still need supervision, to be specific about which parts of their body they should be washing themselves, like their genitals, and which an adult might scrub for them, like their back. They could practice telling an adult to "go away" when they feel something is wrong.

Older children might benefit from a review of rules about privacy. "Taking a bath or a shower with a sibling of the same sex is all right if it is acceptable to both." "No one should be forced into sharing bathroom space." Abused kids need clear boundaries.

Specific rules about bedtime might help a child feel safer too. "No one comes in to say goodnight after the light has been turned out." "Bedtime kisses and hugs are great, but anything else, and the child should get up and go to another adult." Bells on the bedroom door, if it is the child's own room, or some other sound device, might help the child feel more protected.

Nudity that starts after the abuse is <u>not</u> in the best interests of the child. Nudity suggested by a new partner in the home is to be viewed with great suspicion. Taking off clothes does not equal shedding inhibitions, no matter what any "helpful" person says. Children may have difficulty trusting adults who are nude. Nudity may trigger their fear that home isn't safe either. If family nudity has been a fact of life before the abuse, <u>and the abuse occurred outside the family</u> there may be no need to change suddenly.

Teaching about privacy may be necessary. It isn't a good idea to allow a child to watch an adult take a shower, or continually peek at an adult. Staring is an invasion of privacy. Children need to learn that invasions of privacy are a warning sign for them too.

Let's think of some ways you can feel safe at bath time and bedtime.

No one can come in while you are taking a bath unless you say it is okay. You can ask for help washing your back but no one should wash other parts of your body.

No one should come in just to watch or peek.

Goodnight kisses happen before lights out. If someone comes in after that, come tell me.

What would help you feel safer? Would you like bells on your door? a lock? Would you like other rules?

It isn't polite to stare at someone.

Do you know what staring is?

If someone stares or peeks at you when you are undressing, in the bathroom, in your room, in the locker room, please tell me. That is an invasion of your privacy.

Stare Game

What we do is stare at each other until one of us looks away. After we do that a couple of times let's talk about where in our body we feel uncomfortable. My stomach starts to hurt when someone stares at me. Other people blush. Okay ready, let's stare!

FEELING SAFE AGAIN

You may discover, as you talk about self-protection with your child, that she/he is angry with you. Kids often feel let down by the person they thought would protect them or stop the abuse for them. Let the child express that anger toward you. Tell the child that the reason you want to practice safety skills is because you want to do your best to see that the child is protected from any more abuse.

One way to help children be safer is to talk about the ways people get us to do something we might not want to do. Besides the direct power of threats like "Do it or else!" or "I'll hurt your parents (or your puppy) if you don't," there are indirect ways to get people to do things.

The ways people manipulate each other are not confined to sexual abuse, nor are they all bad. They are part of how human beings get along. But the better your child is able to recognize them, the better she/he will be able to resist them when need be.

The family could, as an exercise, discuss one method a week and watch for examples of how others use it. It could be an I Spy game. For example, while waiting in line at the bank, notice how the angry customer is using facial expressions and body movements while making a complaint. Or point out manipulation techniques you see on TV. Together, family members can discuss resisting these techniques. Adults and children alike are vulnerable to these, and can use each other's support in learning how to respond.

The Ways People Manipulate Us:

Method	Lines
Speed	Do it right now! You don't want to miss out!
Defining	You're the kind of child . . . People like you want . . .
Happiness	You would make me happy . . . It would kill your mom . . . Your mom would love it if . . .
Sickness	I'm sick. You have to help me.
Unfair Trade	If you will . . . I will . . . (or won't).
Flattery	You are so good at this. Will you . . .
Guilt	What's the matter—Don't you like me?
Your own good	I want you to know . . . No one else would tell you this.
Labeling	You're so, stupid. You're just a troublemaker!
Overkill	If you don't buy this . . . If you don't do this . . . I'll never come here again.
Gifts	After all I've done for you, the least you can do is . . .
Helplessness	Oh, I didn't mean to do that . . .

People can manipulate us with body language, too. Like crying, or hurt looks, or quivering lower lips.

I remember how much Aunt Jane would cry every time I brought up a problem. Finally I had to say, "I don't want you to cry right now, I want you to listen to me right now".

It helps to stop and figure out what you are feeling. Pay attention to your own feelings.

BEHAVIOR ALERTS

Not only can children be taught to resist manipulation, but they can also learn to recognize some behaviors which signal that something abusive may be starting, or has started.

The Sexual Abuse Warning List comes from comments of sexually abused children (seen at the Sexual Assault Center in Seattle) and describes behaviors that accompanied a gradual drift toward sexual abuse.

You might want to talk about how they are similar and how they are different from the manipulation techniques.

After what your child has been through, it probably makes more sense to talk specifically about sexual abuse, rather than the broader approach of good touch, bad touch. Sexually abused children know that sexual abuse is a lot more than just a bad touch.

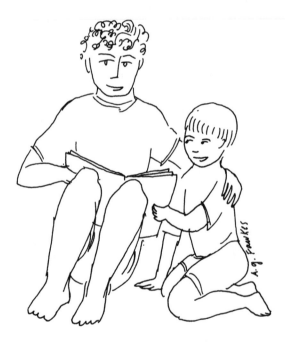

Self-Protection

Sexual Abuse Warning List

Here are some things that other children who have been sexually abused said children could be on the lookout for. Come and tell me if a grown-up is doing any of these things with you:

Treating you differently from other kids: Treating you better than other kids, or being meaner to you. Wanting to spend time alone with you. Making excuses to go places or have others leave. Not letting you have friends or do things that other kids your age do.

Treating you as if you were an adult: Telling you private things, about his wife/your mother. Saying you are different, special, the only one who really understands. Telling you are better than his wife. Or, acting like a kid when he's with you.

Violating your personal space or your privacy: Asking you to do things that involve physical contact, like giving backrubs or washing his back. Accidently-on-purpose brushing against breasts or crotch while wrestling, rubbing his body against yours. Looking at or touching your body and saying it's just to see how you are developing. Putting lotion or ointment on you when there is nothing wrong with you or when your mother or others aren't around. Coming into your room while you are undressed or into the bathroom when you're in there. Not letting you close your bedroom door or the bathroom door. Coming into your bedroom at night. Walking around naked, or accidently-on-purpose letting his robe come apart.

Bribes and secrecy: Giving you special privileges or favors and making you feel obligated. Telling you not to tell your mother or other people about things that happen between you.

Inappropriate talk: Asking questions or making accusations about sexual relations between you and your boy or girlfriend. Teaching "sex education" by showing pornographic pictures, showing you his body or touching your body. Saying sexual things to you about the way you dress. Talking to you about the sexual things he has done.

YOU CAN SAY NO

Maybe your child said no to the abuser, and he didn't stop. Some offenders don't care if a child says no.

In truth, it is very hard for children to say no to any adult. Little permission is given for children to object to adult behavior. For children to say no to advances by adults takes lots of practice. Then it may not stop the offender anyway.

Saying no needs to be treated with a "use it if you can" attitude. If it doesn't work, then children need to move on to the next escape idea: get away, yell, go into the bathroom and lock the door, call someone on the phone, etc.

If someone tries to do this again, you can say no.

Stand tall, square your shoulders, look him in the eye and say "Stop that" or "I don't like that."

Saying no may be too much for you to do. But you could try saying, "I have to go to the bathroom—alone," or "I have to go home now."

TELLING

Perhaps the most important idea to teach children about sexual abuse is to talk about it. And if it happens, tell an adult.

Your child may feel guilty about not telling. You may wonder why she/he didn't tell you. Parents' own feelings of having let the child down tend to come out in the form of "Why didn't you tell!?" Kids tell in their own words, in their own time, when they are capable of it. They do not need to feel badly because they weren't able or didn't know they could tell or didn't know who to tell.

You are already doing a lot of talking with your child about what happened. That is a strong message and encourages them to talk more freely.

It's important for children to know that they can go to someone with questions about sexual abuse. If your child is expecting to be believed and not blamed, she/he might tell you earlier about behavior leading up to abuse. The important job for the child is to tell.

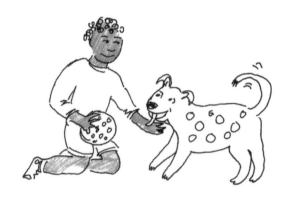

Self-Protection

I'm sorry I didn't believe you. I'll believe you now because I know more about sexual abuse. I'm sorry I was angry. I was angry at Xxxxx, not you. I won't be angry with you if you ever need to tell me it's happening again.

Remember when you had that problem with your bike? I listened and helped then, didn't I? Who else has helped you with different problems?

Name all the people you could tell.

It's a good idea to tell someone about situations similar to the abuse or when someone has asked you to keep a secret or if any behaviors from the sexual abuse warning list come up.

You may think that telling caused too much misery or too many problems. I would have felt worse and much sadder if I hadn't found out what was happening.

Tell your dad or another adult who has helped you since the sexual abuse secret has been out. Who else could you tell? What else could you do?
- Tell the person doing these things that it's not okay and it has to stop and that you have told.
- Realize that he is trying to make you feel guilty, so you won't hold him responsible for what he does.
- Leave the room. Call a friend. Tell your friend. Yell.
- Get help from another adult to see that the behavior stops.

Activities:

Find a storybook and read it together. Stories like "The Little Engine That Could" or other stories of children who have overcome being "one down" are good.

See the book *No More Secrets* (by Adams and Fay, Impact Publishers) for more ideas about preventing sexual abuse.

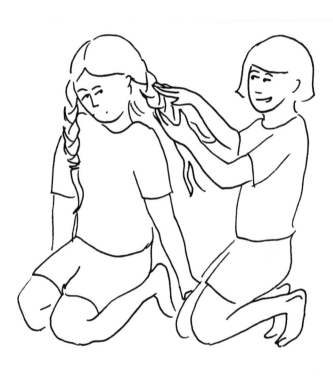

Chapter 9

As Children Grow . . . *"We'll need to talk again"*

"I've never been totally sure how the sexual abuse affected me. My childhood was lonely for a number of reasons, and sometimes the sexual abuse seems pretty minor."

"Only as an adult did I begin to understand how much of what I did was to avoid the pain of the sexual abuse."

HOW LONG DO WE GO ON TALKING ABOUT THIS?

By now you've realized that you can't talk just once about any one part of the abuse and expect a child to understand. You approach the subject from many directions and make times for the child to talk. As children grow, their ability to understand and think about what happened changes. They need continued opportunities to ask questions. Preschoolers understand the abuse differently from the way an eight year old does. A teenager beginning to consider romantic relationships may have one set of concerns then yet another as she/he enters young adulthood.

Parents are children's historians. You help your child understand the continuity of her/his life. At first you may talk when legal actions require preparation, or when your child is frightened, has a nightmare, or asks about the offender. As time passes you may talk about it less, but don't let the subject totally disappear into silence. Your child may be afraid, or may not think to bring it up. You can check every six months or so, then perhaps on the anniversary date of the disclosure.

The sexual abuse may affect you at other times in your life. That's normal.

Let's think of it the same way we think of taking care of our teeth. We don't go to the dentist just once. We go back over the years, to get checked, to have our teeth cleaned, and to get cavities filled. As you grow, you get new teeth. Sometimes there isn't room for those teeth, or other problems come up as part of your growth and change. That's okay when it has to do with your teeth, and that's okay in healing from the abuse.

You can always ask me, no matter how much time has passed, any question you think of, even if you've asked it before.

The sexual abuse began two years ago.

> Do you think about it much?
>
> Do you still have nightmares?
>
> Do you have sexual questions you've been afraid to ask?

Do you worry that maybe you misunderstood and it didn't really happen the way you think it did? That's normal to begin doubting it, even when you know how real it was.

RETURN TO COUNSELING

Consider returning to counseling if your child begins to show the same behavior she/he did after the abuse, such as bedwetting, nightmares, or withdrawal. Each transition stage in a child's life is a time of stress. Symptoms from the abuse may surface again, representing a new need for understanding.

STAGES OF DEVELOPMENT

You may find middle-school age children apparently undisturbed about the sexual abuse, with few questions or concerns. Or you may find that stressful events such as moving or changing schools trigger nightmares related to the abuse. That's normal.

Preadolescence is a particularly difficult transition stage which may be disrupted by abuse. Children in this stage show a number of disturbing characteristics:

- Obsession with physical appearance (I'm so ugly)
- Orientation to the present (Today is all there is)
- Dissatisfaction with parents and school (Why study that?)
- Poor hygiene and poor manners
- Moody behavior (No one will let me be a grown-up)
- Flip-flop of behavior from older to much younger (between 12 and 2, 13 and 3, 15 and 5)
- Rigid morality and a narrow focus on one thing at a time

These normal behaviors can trigger the fear that your child has been damaged more than you thought. However, they are normal. It is not uncommon for children who have been sexually abused to remain in this stage longer than other children.

Children seem to benefit from therapy groups with others their age to share concerns and problem solving. Preadolescence and adolescence may be good times to find such groups.

Times when you are growing and changing may be hard for all of us. Parents and children don't get along all the time even in families without obvious problems.

You can take your time growing up.

I know that you may have questions or doubts that you may not want to ask me about. I'll find a book for you or someone to talk to if you let me know when you want more information.

I know your privacy will be very important to you as you get older. Do you understand the difference between privacy and secrecy? Privacy you keep for yourself. Secrets protect others. Secrets may be okay between you and your friends, but adults shouldn't ask you to keep secrets.

As you get older, you may be afraid to ask questions because you want your privacy. I will try to answer your questions and respect your privacy.

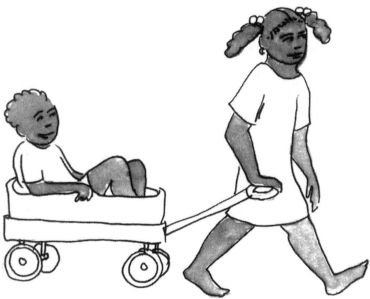

As Children Grow

WARNING SIGNS

At any age these warning signs indicate severe problems for your child. What may not be as obvious is that they may be linked to the past sexual abuse, or suggest recurring victimization. These signs include:

- Running away
- Change in school performance or truancy
- Inability to concentrate
- Delinquent behavior
- Promiscuity
- A frenzy for perfection in school performance
- Intense need for adult approval
- Withdrawal, isolation from friends, living in a fantasy

A child showing any of these behaviors needs your attention and needs help solving the problem.

WHAT ABOUT ADOLESCENCE?

When children reach adolescence, romantic concerns become important. They may be confused about their right to say no, their femininity or masculinity, or about how to set sexual limits. Teens may be unwilling to discuss sexual issues with you, and may respond better to a book written with teens in mind.

It is realistic to mention to your child that some affectionate gestures—kissing, hugging, pats—may be frightening or repulsive. That's normal for anyone who has been sexually victimized.

You may want to discuss the issue of virginity and making choices. All young people should know that past sexual activity—consenting or abusive—need not influence new choices.

Many teenagers don't have severe problems despite all we hear on television about drugs, pregnancy, and runaways. I know that if we keep talking to each other, and we get help when we need it, those problems don't have to happen.

I'm hoping we can work this out so that being a teenager isn't any harder for you than it needs to be.

If you or I run into problems then, there is help we can turn to.

When you get older you may find that some touching reminds you of the sexual abuse —a pat on the butt, or someone coming up behind you and covering your eyes. That's normal. It's okay not to like something, whatever your reason. You don't have to explain.

When you get older I'll ask you some questions again so we can talk about the abuse. I'll probably ask:

Did you feel believed?

What new questions would you like to ask about the abuse now?

Do you think about it much?

YOUR CHILD'S CHOICES

You may want to remind your child that people will not be able to tell that she/he has been abused. The sexual abuse doesn't show in any way. You may want to suggest caution at first when it comes to telling about the abuse. Children may need help in deciding if or when they tell someone.

You may find yourself discouraged about the choices your child makes for dates or friends. She/he may seem to pick the wild kids to run with or find friends who exploit or abuse her/him. Work on building your child's sense that she/he deserves better. It is not helpful to run the friends down.

SETTING LIMITS

Parents remain responsible for setting limits, especially on behavior that directly affects them or younger siblings. If your child insists on activities you consider seductive, dangerous, improper, or risky, you may be unsure about setting limits because of your fear of inhibiting your child or conveying shame. Limits are needed whether the activities are a result of sexual abuse or normal experimentation. The question to ask is, "How would I handle this if the abuse had not taken place?" You may not know the answer, but the question can lead to constructive problem solving.

Children do best when treated as if they are sturdy and capable of repair. As long as you are careful to provide nurturing care, there is no reason to handle problems as if your child is fragile. That tells them they are damaged—the opposite message from the one you want them to have.

You deserve to be treated well.

You deserve to be able to take risks within limits.

I will do everything I can to help. I will get us help if we need it. You will need to do your share, too.

Together we can heal.

Here are some affirmations that might help:

- You can think before you make that rule your own.
- You can trust your feelings to help you to know.
- You can do it your way.
- You can get what you need without suffering.
- You can be a sexual person and still need support, protection, and simple affection.
- It's okay to know who you are.
- You're welcome to come home again.
- I love you.

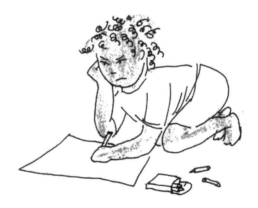

As Children Grow

ARE BOYS AND GIRLS AFFECTED THE SAME WAY?

The effects may be somewhat different, but sexual identity is threatened for both boys and girls. Losing is linked to being less of a man. Femininity is linked to purity. Girls can see themselves as ruined. Secrecy keeps both boys and girls trapped. Boys may feel more alone, more set apart than girls who are victimized. They may be less likely to talk about it. They may have been taught not to cry and to be tough. They may deny that what happened was abuse, thinking of it instead as "being lucky and starting sex early." They may be scared and confused.

Both may ask, "Why me?" Boys may fear they were picked because the offender could "see" something about them. Abuse of boys is more likely to be same-sex abuse, since most offenders are male. Both boys and girls abused by the same sex need reassurance that it has nothing to do with anything the offender saw about them or their future sexual choices.

WILL MY CHILD BECOME AN OFFENDER?

Most children who are abused do not become sex offenders. Although most offenders in treatment programs have been sexually abused, many more of the men abused as children avoid hurting others. Women usually don't become offenders. You have already taken the most important steps by talking, breaking the secrecy, and helping your child learn healthy ways to get her/his needs met.

Some kids who have been abused do some sexually aggressive acting out. If you're not able to stop it, get professional help.

Other boys have been abused—as many as one in seven. That means in every classroom there are one or two other boys who have been abused too. More boys and men have begun to speak out about how hard it is to talk about being sexually abused.

Many children who have been sexually abused <u>do not</u> hurt other children.

The secrecy has been broken. We are talking about it. You've had some help talking about your feelings. All this changes the powerlessness that causes some children to abuse others.

You're no different than any other boy. He picked on you because:
>   You were there.
>   He was looking for a boy your age.
>   He has a problem.

Sometimes even boys can't be in control. All of us—even grown men—sometimes do things we don't want to do (pay taxes, go to funerals).

You're fine just like you are.

There was nothing about <u>you</u> which caused him to pick you.

Right now you are a child—not making sexual choices. That's adult stuff. You have more fun things to think about right now, like games, riding bikes, what flavor ice cream is your favorite.

As you get older, sexual preference develops. The more you heal the more you will be able to make your choices without being influenced by the abuse.

GETTING HELP

If you suspect that your child has become a teenager who may hurt others, the most responsible action is to seek help from a professional who treats adolescent sex offenders. If you are seeking help from someone who tells you, "Boys will be boys" or "It's normal exploration," find another professional.

WE DID EVERYTHING WE COULD

The list of problems linked to sexual abuse is very long. Prostitution, drug or alcohol abuse, early pregnancy, suicide attempts, psychosomatic illnesses, eating disorders, and depression all have been suggested. What isn't known is how many teenagers who develop these problems had help after they disclosed the abuse.

Parents can't fix everything. Children come into the world with very different needs. Some children seem to have the inner resources to survive whatever comes their way. Other children do okay with adequate help and resources. Some children need more help, more than society is prepared to provide.

There are limits to what parents can do. As children grow up, they can begin to take the responsibility for healing.

Many adults, sexually abused as children, have healed after years of trauma.

No is Not Enough, (by Adams and Fay, Impact Publishers), has many ideas about how to talk to your children as they reach adolescence.

Sexual abuse happens to lots of kids, and has for a long time. Only some of those who are abused grow up to hurt others. They are usually the ones who don't tell anyone or get any help.

If you wonder if something isn't okay for the other person, please ask me, or ___.

Sometimes kids who don't learn new ways to feel powerful again, or in control, do what was done to them to feel better. But you don't need to do that. We'll talk about this again soon.

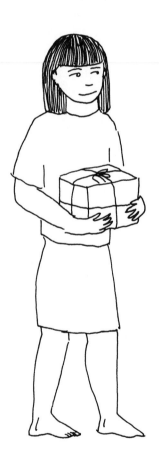

Chapter 10

Moving On . . . *"It's better now"*

"Forgive him you say?
He who did the unthinkable
and then lied and made my child cry.

Never! I spit. Never!
I want him hung, strung,
I want him to suffer days
as nights
my child screamed.
As many as I waited for justice.
He should burn—Forgive him?
Hah!—you hear?"

But . . . You're not kidding are you?
You say my anger is burning a hole in my days.
Tearing the fabric of my life,
Is a knife turning on me
and my child."

"Can't I just forget?"

FINDING AN END

Three months, six months, a year from now, you will realize hours have passed without the abuse crossing your mind. You've laughed at a joke, or enjoyed a day in the sunshine. You begin to believe you will not always be buried under the bitter, angry, and cynical feelings. To continue to free yourself, you need to reclaim the energy you are putting into hopes for apologies or revenge, and find a way to rebuild faith and trust.

If forgetting means separating and letting go, that may be enough. Forgiveness is often suggested too early. Some people cannot be forgiven, only released from your concern. Don't let anyone push you into forgiveness. It may be helpful to you and your child to let go of resentment.

Naming Exercise

Let's print Xxxxx's name on this piece of paper and put it in this can and put it away. You could draw a picture of him too, and we'll just put him away for a while.

If you are still really mad, we could burn the picture, or rip it into a thousand pieces. Do you want to do that?

FREE FROM ANGER

You may need to let go of anger at others before you are free to move on:

- Your husband (why didn't he help, understand?)
- The child's father (why did he fight me instead of helping?)
- Your mother (why does she always blame me?)
- A prosecutor (how could he have plea bargained?)

You may be able to excuse some people through an awareness that they reacted from fear or ignorance. They may have apologized for their inability to act. But others may continue only to ignore your pain. You need to be independent of their actions for your own recovery. Continuing to want something from them leaves them in control. When you let go of expectations of them, you can continue on your road.

SELF-FORGIVENESS

You may blame yourself for what happened to your child. The offender is responsible for the abuse, but some people think parents can stop it. If you share that judgment, you need to find a way to forgive yourself. Sometimes other life problems interfere with a parent's ability to provide protection to a child. Alcoholism in the family, past childhood sexual abuse, care of an elderly parent or a sick sibling, poverty and unemployment, violent abuse—all are factors that can make it more difficult.

Forgiving yourself may mean getting help for your own problems, or changing some circumstances of your life. Promise yourself you need not suffer all your life for what you feel were your shortcomings. If you need to take action to feel better, do so, but put a time limit on whatever you do.

Who are you still mad at?
   Me?
   Grandma?
   The person who told?
   Someone else?

What would you like him (daddy, your uncle, the baby-sitter) to say to you? Would you like him to say:
   I'm sorry. I know I hurt you. It must have been hard to keep a secret. I know I was wrong.

What do you wish would happen to him/her?

Sometimes even when someone does something to us that isn't right or fair, we still have to let go of being mad at them so we can move on to new friends, games, and better feelings.

FAITH

No matter what your formal religious affiliation, your faith in an orderly world has been shaken. You may have known that children were sexually abused, but you hoped, prayed, or just assumed that it wouldn't happen to your children.

Our society is based on the notion that if you work hard, you will be rewarded. If bad things happen to you, you must have been bad somehow. Most of us know that isn't true, but it allows us to feel in control. Sometimes people make unthinking remarks which contribute to the pain:

"God is punishing you for something."

"God doesn't give us burdens we can't bear."

"You must be wrong. You are accusing a God-fearing man."

Just when you need the support of the community, you may feel betrayed. Somehow you will need to overcome the alienation and find a place within the community. Some religious communities are working to provide better comfort to families in which sexual abuse has occurred.

You and your child need to find a new version of the world which makes sense to you. You need to answer the question, "How can people do something this hurtful to others?" in a way that doesn't condemn all men, all teenagers, or all of any group. You will need to accept the impossibility of protecting your child totally. You do what you can to provide supervision, information, follow any rules about secrecy given by a counseling program, and indicate your willingness to listen to your child. That is the best you can do.

Let's talk about luck.

Luck means we aren't totally in control of what happens to us. Sometimes good things happen, sometimes bad.

Good luck is being in the right place at the right time without planning to be. Being at the bus stop early when the bus happens to come early—that's partly luck.

Bad luck means being in the wrong place at the wrong time, without planning to be. Being outside when a sudden rainstorm soaks you. Walking by a yard where a biting dog has just gotten loose. That's bad luck for you. That is not your fault.

You can't depend on luck. Taking care of yourself as well as you can keeps you safer. Doing the best we can helps our luck be good. We can't stay trapped because we are afraid of bad luck.

Some actions by people are not under our control. Some people are hurtful to others because they were hurt. Some are hurtful because they don't know they are hurting others. Some like to hurt other people because they think they have the right.

It doesn't always make sense.

It's never okay to hurt people the way you were hurt.

CONTINUING CONTACT

People may suggest you forgive the offender. Certainly you cannot pardon him, or excuse what he did. If you never see him, you may be able to release your wish for revenge and forget him.

Rebuilding faith, and learning how to trust again, will be easier if you are not forced to have continuing contact with the offender. Allowing the person back into your life should happen only if you and your child have healed, and the other person has shown he is doing something to change—not just promised, but actually doing. He should acknowledge responsibility that neither you nor your child was to blame, and that the abuse has caused both you and your child pain. You and your child should control the timing of this. Don't let your child be pressured into accepting an apology.

The offender should not be allowed in your life because he or anyone else asked or demanded it, but sometimes you have no choice. The abuser may be the child's father, who continues to have visitation rights, an uncle or grandparent who continues to be at family gatherings, or a neighbor's teenage child who is still in the neighborhood.

The agony of not being able to protect your child totally or being torn between protecting your child and continuing a relationship with someone you love makes any final resolution much more difficult. The difficulty makes outside help necessary. You will need all your strength and flexibility to remain available to your child, and able to help when she/he needs it.

Box Closure

Let's keep all the papers and pictures you draw and maybe even this book in this special box. When we don't have any court dates, or counseling appointments, and we are going to just live normally for a while, we will put the box away. We can tie a strong piece of twine around it, and just put it away. But we can take it out and look through it any time you want to.

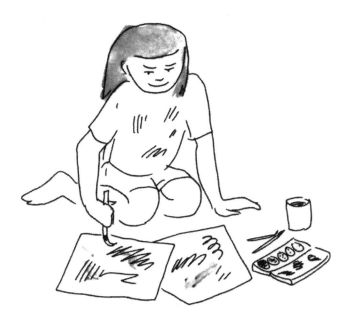

SOCIAL ACTION

Society gives two messages about child sexual abuse:

"It is a horrid, repulsive crime against children."

and

"Children really like it. It is adults who make it bad."

Preventing sexual abuse will take a societal effort:

- Young sex offenders must be identified and treated.
- Abuse victims must be identified and treated.
- The societal norms that allow men to rationalize and deny the harm they are doing to children must be changed.
- The criminal justice system must be modified to accommodate child victims.

It can be very healing to find the people in your community who are working on these issues and join them. As you look for a group to work with, look for those who acknowledge multiple causes of child sexual abuse and don't blame any particular group of people as the cause. You will discover other parents using their anger in constructive ways to change the way child sexual abuse is tolerated and allowed to continue.

SELECTED RESOURCES

A VERY TOUCHING BOOK: For Little People and for Big People, by Jan Hindman. McClure-Hindman Books, 1983. Available in bookstores or from:

> Alexandria Associates
> (541) 889-8938.

A colorful cartoon-illustrated picture book for children that uses humor and honesty to open communication with children about sexual abuse, privacy and their bodies. Used in both prevention and treatment of sexual abuse.

THE MOTHER'S BOOK: How to Survive the Molestation of Your Child, by Carolyn M. Byerly, 2nd ed. Kendall-Hunt Publishing Company, 1992. Available in bookstores or from:

> The Center for Prevention of Sexual
> and Domestic Violence
> 936 N. 34th Street, Suite 200
> Seattle, WA 98103
> (206) 634-1903 Fax (206) 634-0115
> or on the web at http://www.cpsdv.org/

A supportive book for the mother; contents include cultural issues faced by mothers of color, common religious issues surrounding incest, and the criminal justice process.

SEXUAL ABUSE PREVENTION: A Course of Study for Teenagers, by Rebecca Voelkel-Haugen and Rev. Marie M. Fortune. The United Church Press, 1992. Available from The Center for Prevention of Sexual and Domestic Violence (see address above).

A curriculum for teen religious education classes. Six sessions provide information ranging from the facts and myths of sexual assault to media messages about women, men and relationships.

NO MORE SECRETS: Protecting Your Child from Sexual Assault,
by Caren Adams and Jennifer Fay. Impact Publishers, 1981. Available
in bookstores or from:

> Impact Publishers
> PO Box 910
> San Luis Obispo, CA 93406
> (805) 543-5911 Fax (805) 543-4093
> or by email at 74133.303@compuserve.com

A practical, non-judgmental guide for talking with children under
twelve about sexual abuse and how they might protect themselves. Emphasizes the parent's role in prevention.

**WHEN THE BOUGH BREAKS: A Helping Guide for Parents of
Sexually Abused Children,** by Aphrodite Matsakis. New Harbinger
Publications, 1991. Available in bookstores or from:

> New Harbinger Publications
> 5674 Shattuck Avenue
> Oakland, CA 94609-1662
> (510) 652-0215
> or by email at nhhelp@newharbinger.com

Includes chapters on what to do when your child is suicidal, when
to consider hospitalization, when hospitalization is necessary and
what to do afterwards, as well as a resource list of organizations
helpful to sexual abuse survivors and their families.

**COURAGE TO HEAL: A Guide For Women Survivors of Child
Sexual Abuse,** by Ellen Bass and Laura Davis. HarperCollins, 1997.
Available in bookstores or from:

> HarperCollins
> (800) 331-3761
> or on the web at http://www.harpercollins.com/

For adults, this life-affirming and supportive guide answers the
question, what happens next?: once the childhood sexual abuse

has been squarely faced, how does one heal? Quotes from the experiences of hundreds of adult survivors. An updated and revised edition.

ALLIES IN HEALING: When the Person You Love Was Sexually Abused as a Child, by Laura Davis. HarperCollins, 1991. Available in bookstores or from HarperCollins (see address above).

The book answers the questions most often asked by partners and extended families of survivors of child sexual abuse. Shares the stories, struggles and triumphs of partners in the process of healing.

FREE OF THE SHADOWS: Recovering from Sexual Violence, by Caren Adams and Jennifer Fay. New Harbinger Publications, 1989. Discounts available to rape crisis centers, shelters, and victims assistance programs. Available in bookstores or from New Harbinger Publications (see address above).

Step-by-step help for teens or adults who have been raped, with notes for family and friends. Provides ideas for how to get through the days and months after the sexual violence and offer hope about the healing process.

WHAT IS SEXUAL ABUSE?

Legal definitions of sexual abuse differ from state to state and may differ from the following ones. Listed here are forms of abuse, such as kissing, which may not be illegal but are still abusive if they are leading to further contact.

One definition of sexual abuse is that it is forced, tricked, or coerced sexual behavior between a young person and an older person, with the understanding that "force" is always present in any sexual abuse.

The types of sexual behavior may include:

Exhibitionism, in which an adult exposes his genitals to a child. In a family context in which nudity and privacy norms may vary, if the intent is the adult's sexual gratification, or intimidation of the child, then it is abusive.

Voyeurism, in which an adult watches a child undress, bathe, or use the bathroom. Again the intent is important, since there are many situations in which adults appropriately monitor children during these activities. Children can often tell you that "something is funny."

Kissing, in which the adult gives the child lingering or intimate kisses, especially on the mouth and perhaps with the adult's tongue stuck in the child's mouth.

Fondling, in which an offender touches, caresses, or rubs a child's genitals or breasts, or has the child similarly touch his body. Rubbing a child's back, head, or other "nonsexual" part of the body may be abusive if its intent is to engage the child in a situation that will lead to actual sexual behavior.

Fellatio or cunnilingus, in which an adult forces a child to have oral-genital contact with him.

Vaginal or anal intercourse, in which the adult penetrates the child's vaginal or anal opening with a finger, penis, or object.

Pornography, when children are shown material depicting graphically specific sexual acts between adults, adults and children, or children as part of a situation in which abuse takes place, or pornographic pictures or film may be taken of them.

For further information see *A Look at Child Sexual Abuse,* a booklet by Jon R. Conte, available from the National Committee for Prevention of Child Abuse, 332 South Michigan Ave. Suite 1600, Chicago, IL 60604. (312) 663-3520.

OFFENDER INFORMATION: "HOW COULD HE?"

Most likely the person who victimized your child was either an acquaintance or a family member, not a stranger. One of the most puzzling questions about sexual victimization of children is why adults engage in a behavior that is illegal and considered so unthinkable by most people. Although there are many relatively simple answers such as "he was abused himself," when examined they fail to explain why one person abuses others while another doesn't. Incest was considered a separate category of abuse until it was learned that nearly half of incest offenders also abused outside the family. No profile or simple statement adequately answers this question. What is known is that:

Offenders will offend again unless they get specialized treatment, and maintain a careful awareness of the circumstances that could lead to a new offense.

Offenders cannot follow through on good intentions or genuine remorse without help from outside the family.

Treatment of offenders is very difficult. It requires extensive specialized training, information, and skills.

Offenders do not fit any profile. They may be upstanding members of the community, even people with strong religious and moral beliefs. Some offenders are teenagers.

Offenders will deny and minimize their behavior toward children. If pressured, they may admit some part of their behavior but offer excuses:
My wife doesn't give me sex any more.
It didn't hurt the child.
I was drunk.
She seduced me.
She made it up.

It is probably wisest to view sex offenders as never "cured," but recovering, through outside intervention, support, treatment, and continued watchfulness.

ABOUT THE AUTHORS

Caren Adams, M.A., began in 1973 to assist sexual assault victims and their families, and to explore ways to prevent rape and sexual abuse.

Jennifer Fay, M.A., has specialized in sexual assault prevention since 1979, when she wrote "He Told Me Not to Tell," one of the first booklets to encourage parents to talk to their children about sexual assault.

Both authors draw on years of experience in the anti-rape movement as crisis counselors and in the creation of programs for social change.

This is the fourth book by Adams and Fay aimed at lessening the impact of sexual violence in our lives. Their other books include *No More Secrets*, *No is Not Enough* (co-authored with Jan Loreen-Martin), and *Free of the Shadows*.